BORDERLINE PERSONALITY DISORDER

Spouse Has Borderline Personality Disorder

(Everything You Need to Know About
Borderline Personality Disorder)

Gabriel Hopper

Published By Gabriel Hopper

Gabriel Hopper

*Borderline Personality Disorder: Spouse Has Borderline
Personality Disorder (Everything You Need to Know About
Borderline Personality Disorder)*

ISBN 978-1-77485-423-5

Legal & Disclaimer

The information contained in this book is not designed to replace or take the place of any form of medicine or professional medical advice. The information in this book has been provided for educational and entertainment purposes only.

The information contained in this book has been compiled from sources deemed reliable, and it is accurate to the best of the Author's knowledge; however, the Author cannot guarantee its accuracy and validity and cannot be held liable for any errors or omissions. Changes are periodically made to this book. You must consult your doctor or get professional medical advice before using any of the suggested remedies, techniques, or information in this book.

TABLE OF CONTENTS

Introduction

There's always been a stigma associated with those who are deemed mentally sick. They are often portrayed socially to be "crazy", "hysteric" or even those who do not have the necessary discipline to create their lives better. People aren't aware the fact that people diagnosed with mental illness face a challenge that is real and they're experiencing a very difficult experience.

Mental illness does not spare anyone child, teenager or adults, not to mention older people. It is likely that you have a parent, friend or sibling or coworker with the condition. If a loved one suffers from it, it affects the nature of relationships that we have.

Sometimes, psychiatric issues can be so severe that they can wreak chaos on the whole family simply because the people aren't aware enough about them, or how to manage it. If these issues aren't dealt with in a timely manner, they could lead to a devastating cycle of hurt and blame.

The most frequent mental disorder is called borderline personality disorder (BPD) that affects about 2 percent from the American population every year. It is defined by the inability to sustain steady relationships in the family and reckless behavior. That is why it is frequently called emotional instability personality disorder or emotional intensity disorder in addition to other. The symptoms of borderline personality disorder generally manifest in the early years of childhood or adolescence however it may develop later in life for other people. BPD is often associated with suicide and self-harm, however, if diagnosed early and treated, the outlook is very good.

If you're interested in learning more about the disorder known as borderline personality You've come to the right location. Through this book, you'll discover all the aspects of this mysterious , yet widespread illness.

Chapter 1: Understanding Your Relationship

Before you can get back to your senses You must be aware of the nature of your relationship, which includes the person you were with as well as the reason you were doing it, as well as the reason why it was bound to fail right from the beginning. Why is this breakup causing so much pain more than other breakups? We will discuss this in this article. The answer is extremely complex , and there are several aspects to be considered.

If you have come across this program, then likely, you've searched the internet for info on borderline personality disorder to try to comprehend the issues. Maybe you had an epiphany moment similar to mine when I realized I was dating a disordered person. Perhaps you've been experiencing pain that is unbearable for a long time and then finally realized you were in a relationship with someone emotional unstable, after looking for answers that you might discover.

However, I am not a licensed doctor and I'm not able to determine the cause of your ex. And neither can you. Whatever name you choose to use to your ex you're clearly in an unimaginable amount of emotional turmoil. If you didn't, you wouldn't be experiencing the pain that you're experiencing right now looking for answers or this guide on the subject.

The majority in this article will provide the links to additional sources and articles from experts in the field of personality Disorders and behavior. Understanding and reading them is the very first step towards getting yourself back to health. Since it's easy to fall into the process of understanding I suggest you only read only one article per day , at the most. They require reading them over and over in order to absorb them fully. Too many readings in a short time will prove to be ineffective.

Who was your ex-partner?

No matter if your ex-partner was classified as having borderline personality Disorder or displayed traits that indicated they were in a relationship with a unstable person, or else you wouldn't suffer this much.

In the aftermath of an breakup with a disordered person, our instinctual response is to discover everything that we can about them. We would like to know more about their behaviour and explain it in our heads.

When we know the person we were with in the first place, we can free ourselves from the guilt and guilt that comes with the breakup and relationship. There's nothing wrong with this and it's an essential step on the direction of recovery.

What I observed while browsing forums for those who are in a relationship that is abusive People tend to focus on the way they can understand their partner. They frequently ask the same questions and then receive slightly different answers to the same question.

Obsessed with understanding your partner's needs can hinder you from recovering or learning lessons from this devastating event. While we would like to spend time in this stage however, we must get to a better understanding of ourselves. At some point researching more about Borderline/Narcissistic/Histrionic Personality Disorder will serve you no good. There's a minimum threshold for understanding the behavior of your ex and there's nothing gain in attempting to surpass it. The most effective approach is to give up the fact that you'll never fully comprehend their destructive behaviour.

While it's important to be aware of the behaviour of your ex however, I believe it's essential to learn about your own motivations and why you felt drawn to your ex first. Therefore, I chose to keep this section brief since it is likely that you have already spent many hours studying personality disorders on the internet.

What made you fall in love with an emotionally troubled person? What does this mean about you?

"Someone who is truly positive, confident self-confidence Self is not a person who gets confused with someone who has a personality disorder. Any person who is not in this category has unresolved pain in the core and shame that has accumulated from childhood. The personality disordered person triggers early trauma to your feelings of love and worth. That's why the reason you're reading this."

This is the most vital to learn about yourself as it will help you understand your identity and why you ended up being this way. Although it's easy to describe someone as an emotionally dysfunctional spouse (and it is likely that they are) and then fall back to an attitude of victimization however, one must ask what led you to end being with them? It is a fact that you attract the person you portray.

Did your mother suffer from depression as you grew as a child? Did she suffer from major mood swings, and did you do everything you could to make her feel more relaxed and content? Additionally, do you frequently feel like you're accountable for the mood of others, from relatives and friends to your spouse?

It Is a common pattern among codependents and those who are more likely to be attracted by emotionally abusive partners who have personalities disorders (BPD, HPD, NPD). From a young age, you may have been placed in situations where your mom was unable to provide you with the tender care, love and affection you required to grow into an emotionally well-balanced adult.

Instead of nourishing your mother, she likely relied on you to provide her with emotional support which is why you were taught unintentionally that your happiness was contingent on hers. It was taught to you by your parents that to be really happy, you had to do all you could to spare your mom from suffering and sorrow. This dysfunctional relationship has been the basis for all other relationships that you have ever had.

In the midst of all this you could be thinking that you are the parent, rather than them being your parents. You might are tempted to offer others advice instead of focussing on yourself. If you have a family member or friend who isn't completely supportive of your advice, you may become angry and take it personal. Do you feel like this?

Like you did when an infant with your mom likely, you were drawn to the idea that you could repair or save your loved one. The notion of being loved was your personal gauge of self-worth. These behavior patterns are now in the cover of what is now referred to as Codependency.

What is the cause of your inexplicably discomfort?

You can tell that the degree of suffering you're experiencing is unlike anything you've ever experienced. Personally, I felt exhausted, and unable to complete even the most basic tasks. The grief I felt resulted in me losing my job.

It is likely that your ex has brought about the trauma and shame from your childhood which you've carried for the rest of your life. The separation from your ex brought this issue to the surface However, you should know that this hurt has nothing to be related to your ex.

Many of you have experienced similar discomfort when you were young children, most likely between the ages of one to three. Most of the time your mother didn't show you how to cope with the pain, which is why you had to handle it by yourself.

You've mastered the art of not feeling pain due to the fact that you were not taught to do it effectively. Instead, your instinct is to think about the pain and assign significance to it. As you progress through the course, you will begin learn to truly feel the pain and will realize that it isn't going to cause you to die!

Why is reuniting with your ex the most awful thing you could do?

While your mind is racing and you are looking for a solution to ease the agonizing pain you're currently experiencing, it might be tempting to go back together with your ex. You always tell yourself that returning to them will help make the pain disappear. This could not be further than the fact.

Certain, you'll experience an initial feeling of peace if you go back with your ex-partner, however, soon the stress you felt before will resurface with the emotional physical abuse, tensions of push and pull, and the failure to maintain the healthy relationship will be brought back with full force. You'll be getting ready for more severe hurt later on.

In a way that is sad the majority individuals who've been with emotionally abusive individuals have a numbing addiction to suffering. We are thriving off the experience and are able to fill us with raw emotions of life that we've never experienced otherwise. Like applying a band-aid on a deep cut that requires stitching your hurt has nothing to do with be related to your past.

If you have broken up with your ex and would love to be with your ex, your instinct told you it was time to break up because of reasons. Consider the times that you've had in your life where your gut feelings were so powerful that you couldn't ignore it. Maybe you were worried that you'd be dismissed out of work? You felt uneasy having a conversation with a specific individual, but your instinct was telling you something was not right.

Our instinct for survival is a vital element of our biology. It's no accident that when our species evolved we developed an instinct that can aid us in our survival. Don't be fooled, your instincts aren't always leading you wrong. We, as codependents, have been taught to avoid our own feelings and try to analyze things in a way that isn't helpful even though the right answers are being provided to us by our bodies! Doesn't that sound ridiculous? This was the case for me as I was taught to do this by one of the most renowned experts in childhood trauma.

If you broke up with your ex, or they broke up with you or you are in the middle of an abusive relationship were you to have followed your gut and acted accordingly, you wouldn't be reading this book today. It is likely that your gut has been telling you to stay alert throughout the entire time.

Chapter 2: Getting Yourself Back

No contact

The sinister and vicious breakup/reconciliation cycles that often result from dating a borderline individual can inflict tremendous damage upon you. The earlier you adhere to the strict no-contact policy that are laid out in the following, the quicker you will begin to heal yourself. Don't assume that you're strong enough or possess the determination to avoid your ex's message if they decide to contact you. I've read about individuals who have heard about their ex-partners many years later and then being sucked in a vicious cycle. You won't be among the others!

Now your body is craving acceptance of your partner. It would like to know you're still wanted since you may have been in an intimate relationship with someone who you believed could be "the perfect one" or the person you would love to be with. It is possible that you are wondering why your ex suddenly cease communication with you after they've told you that you're your love in their lives. How can they turn off a light?

Rememberthat your ex's emotional power is like the capacity of a 3-year old. They can't feel genuine affection because they did not have the chance to grow emotionally. It's a tough concept to take in however, you have to be able to accept it so that you can understand who you were actually dating.

In addition, you must be aware that there is no way to heal your ex-partner or repair your relationship. Any attempt to reach your ex-partner who has been unable to contact you will result in their own selfish needs.

Breaking up is never simple, but it's much more difficult now because of the prevalence on social networks. Social media could keep you in a constant state of mind over the person you love. If you're like me was, you'll need to monitor every move that your ex makes to find out if they're in a relationship with someone else or whether they're moving on with their lives. You'll be looking for any indication that your ex has you in their thoughts. This seems like self-inflicted suffering for me and we're going to make sure that you do not commit this again.

If you decide to follow only one section of this manual make it this section. Nothing can guide your recovery in a better way than following the guidelines for no contact I provided below. You must adhere to all of them!

Phone - I recommend blocking their phone telephone number, or switching their numbers to your own. I'm a big lover of the latter option because this way, you don't keep their number on your phone. Additionally, every when you attempt to message her, you'll end up messaging yourself instead.

Facebook - unfriend your ex and seriously consider blocking them. I'm a big advocate of blocking them since you are still able to view their profile even after you unfriend them. Do yourself a favor and stop. If you absolutely have to removed, you can remove Facebook for a few days until you can get your feet back.

Instagram - unfollow your ex and set your Instagram account to private. People with borderline disorders are known for their extreme jealousy and episodes of intense rage. If necessary, you can delete this app off your device at present.

Email Block their email. We'd like to shut all doors.

How to deal with depression

Do you wake up in the morning seem very difficult? After your breakup, you could feel depressed, anxious or sleeplessness, getting up, having nightmares and even an inability to eat. I have experienced all of these and found the daily grind to be extremely stressful.

To restore and recover to an emotional health state, it is necessary to boost the depression level that you're in to a level that is manageable. Here are some supplements and suggestions to fight it.

Contact your physician in case you experience any adverse side effects due to the following supplements, and stop taking it right away.

Inositol Powder

We'd like to decrease the frequency of the mind chatter you're experiencing. If you're constantly thinking about your ex and are not being able to think of other things You may be displaying signs of OCD that is aggressive. OCD.

Inositol Powder has been shown to be a positive effect immediately in treating OCD. It reduces how much obsessive thoughts that you are engaged in throughout your day. Since this is an naturally-occurring chemical and is present in numerous food items people consume on a regular basis, there is little to no negative side negative effects.

Inositol is available in powder or pills. It is recommended to buy powdered forms which I discovered on Amazon at $15. My suggestion is Jarrow Formula's .

Begin with a dose of 1/2 teaspoon twice daily. For consumption it, mix the powder with a tiny amount of juice or water and drink. It will have a mildly sweet flavor , and isn't too difficult to take in. If you're experiencing any adverse reactions take it off immediately and speak with your doctor.

St. John's Wort

St. John's wort is an herb. The leaves and flowers can be used to create medicines.

St. John's wort is often used to treat depression, as well as conditions that can are associated with depression like fatigue, anxiety weight loss, nausea and sleeplessness. There is strong scientific proof that it is beneficial for mild to moderate depression.

There is St. John's wort at any drugstore, however my recommendation is to stay clear of brands like Nature's Way. The store-branded offerings are also available. St. John's Wort include those offered by Trader Joe's and Whole Foods are my top choices.

Depending on the mg of each capsule, I suggest taking 600mg daily in the morning to kick with if you're suffering from symptoms of mild to moderate depression. This is usually equivalent to taking a few capsules daily.

Be aware of how you feel when using this dose. If you're experiencing problems sleeping, cut the dosage to 300 mg per day and check the way you are feeling. If you continue to experience adverse effects, you should stop taking it and talk to an expert physician.

A few of you may be able to handle more of a dose. If you are feeling good early in the day but you notice a decline during the afternoon, feel at ease taking a few additional capsules at 2 or 3 pm. Like we said, you should reduce the dosage if it disrupts your sleeping patterns.

If you're experiencing extreme depression or suicidal ideas, you must consult an emergency physician right away! Most likely, you'll require a more aggressive treatment, such as an antidepressant prescription.

Water

Hydration is an integral part of both your physical and mental well-being. If you're not drinking at least 64 oz of water on a regular basis then you'll be feeling tired, anxious, and maybe even depressed!

To make this process easier for you, take 20oz of fluids upon the first day of your life. It will get your day started in the right way and will give you energy throughout the day.

Sleep

A lot of you have or are likely to experience difficulties sleeping. Perhaps you are experiencing intense nightmares or wake up at the end of the night, and are unable to go back to sleep. In the initial month following my breakup I could not rest for more than 4 hours per night.

Depression can be exacerbated by sleep problems and make the seemingly unsolvable crisis that you're facing more difficult. I've had the worst nightmares after waking in the early hours of the morning from the nightmare, and in a state of denial and unable to go to sleep.

Exercise

In the present day there is no way I'll need to talk about the benefits of fitness and how it helps in the fight against depression and stop it from occurring. Because of the traumatizing character of the break-up you should be operating at full speed.

My favourite forms of exercise include yoga and rock climbing. I've found that climbing helps me to be completely focused and divert my thoughts for a while and yoga allows me to relax and calm my mind for hours. Additionally I am able to sleep better after a yoga session.

Get regular exercises (4plus days per week) as part of your daily routine and you'll see immediate results.

Coping with Pain

If you have found yourself drawn to someone who has Borderline Personality traits, then you've likely suffered from the pain of your whole life. As we've said before the fact that you were not taught to handle the pain you felt when you were a kid.

In order to endure these uneasy sensations, which could seem like they're going be a death sentence at times, you've probably turned to other methods to cope, such as the use of alcohol, drugs, sexual pornography, binge eating extreme exercise, thinking too much and over-working, and, with no doubt the possibility of a relationship.

To grow into an emotionally complete person You must develop the capacity to deal with all kinds of emotions, which includes pain and anxiety, without having to resort to external measures of relief. This section will help you achieve this.

Deep Breathing to cope with Pain

If you're anything like I was, you can't endure the pain of a typhoon like the pain you is probably affecting you today. The natural reaction is likely to dwell on this pain, and attempt to connect some meaning to it. The thoughts I had after my ex-wife shut me out were:

* Nobody will ever again love me.

* I'll never find anyone as great as my former one was.

* My ex-partner left me due to the fact that I'm unlucky and failed.

* I'm so stupid for having me get in a relationship with an ex.

* I'm not able to accomplish anything correctly.

* I'm not the best person to be.

However, the urge to believe this could cause prolonged periods of depression that are self-inflicted. When I was in the midst of my most intense times of suffering following the separation, I'd frequently have depression-like episodes that would last up to three days. I didn't realize of the fact that I had made it more difficult than they needed to be.

And the worst part is the fact that you're likely not aware of the fact of what you're doing! I'm sure I didn't. This is fine and we will end the cycle of connecting meaning to pain. From now on when you feel discomfort, I would like you to follow these steps:

Deep Breathing Exercise

Take a deep breath and count to five, and then slowly exhale for five minutes. Keep your eyes on your breathing while you're doing this to put aside the thoughts you naturally do. It can also help to close your eyes. Do this for at 5 minutes at a minimum If that's too much, then try for two minutes to begin with.

When you're breathing deeply Rub any part of your body that feel discomfort. My experience was typically in the upper region of my chest, in the vicinity of the solar plexus.

Note how the pain dramatically diminishes after you have completed this workout? The results are immediateand you'll be able to feel a soothing sensation throughout the region where you felt pain. It will take efforts and time on your part, especially at the beginning! It is important to resist the urge to get inside your head and try to rationalize your feelings of pain. The thoughts that come up in your mind do not have any truth and can lead to self-destructive thoughts.

When you have done this exercise several times, you'll notice the pain diminishing every time. It is because you are developing your emotional muscle and your capacity to feel and sit through painful emotions. As time passes you'll begin to recognize that these feelings aren't likely to harm you.

Friends and Family

In this difficult time of your lives, it's vital to surround yourself with people who will help you. If you're anything like me, you may have lost touch with friends you loved and even some family members because of what you were doing in your friendship.

Although you may be uncomfortable, is the time to connect with your circle of friends, particularly the ones with whom you've lost contact. A genuine friend will feel your pain and sympathize with the situation you're experiencing and will not make you feel guilty for your withdrawal. Some might express anger however, the majority will accept your apology.

As a note to be cautious, you should mindful who you talk about your breakup. If you find that some family members or friends get angry with you and are unable understand the reason why your breakup is affecting your life so much it is best to stop talking to them about the breakup.

Every individual in your world is one another. Some people aren't able to be good listeners and give them the support you require. Do your best to not engage in disputes with them instead, opt to refrain from talking to them about the breakup.

Friends or family members who are unsupportive generally suggest that you "snap off of the situation", "get over it" or "move ahead". If you have heard these or similar statements from someone, you've discovered that you are unable to confide in them. Interacting with them can only make you feel worse than you are already.

Most often, those who do not support each other are not able to accept their own emotions. Don't be surprised by the ones who urge you to drink alcohol or to do drugs together!

It is crucial to seek out compassionate people who are capable of empathizing with your and stay clear of those who would put you down.

Chapter 3: Rebuilding Yourself

Maintaining your routine

If you're feeling the same way as I was following my breakup, getting out of bed could appear like a daunting task. I would usually lay in my bed for hours thinking about negative thoughts, and wondering whether my life was filled with reason or significance.

In this period it is vital that you be consistent with your daily routine. Avoid any urge to take a break from work, no matter when you are unable to stop at your desk and you aren't able to concentrate.

If you choose to stay home and do not continue with your routine every day You are creating the conditions for a long-lasting period of depression. Instead of the use of will power which I'm not a big person to do, I would rather to use a reward system.

Every night, I would like you to record three things you're planning to complete the following day. They should be small items, such as showering at the beginning of the day, going to work, or having 2 glasses of water once you awake. The more insignificant the more important! Before you get to bed I would like you to say loudly:

"I am extremely happy with myself for having an early shower before going to work and drinking 2 glasses of water once I got up!"

Alongside the daily rewards routine I would suggest scheduling your week in advance. Every Saturday and Sunday, take a seat to your planner and map out what you're going to do throughout the day. It is crucial to plan out your weekends and evenings, because they are especially stressful times in which your mind wanders the most. In addition, you usually spent those times with your partner.

Activities

Breakups can be painful and challenging and have been proven scientifically to cause physical discomfort. The process of healing from a breakup someone who is emotionally abusive, but, it's an impossible endeavor. More than ever, it's the right time to concentrate on your own health and seek out healthy avenues to express yourself.

A large part of recovery is recovering yourself. For me, it was yoga, climbing rocks, as well as playing the guitar. When I was climbing, doing yoga , or playing guitar, I could completely concentrate and never think of any other thing.

If you're interested in hobbies have been slack because of your relationship, you can try to force yourself to pick them up. Remember, you used take pleasure in these activities and I am nearly certain that you will once you get back into these activities.

It is not about watching tv or movies. I suggest you choose one that you're interested in. If you're unable to find one, then explore different options until you have discovered the one you like. Here are some ideas to get started:

You can take an instructor in yoga.

• Take an introduction to rock climbing class if have a gym in your area.

* Join an Improv comedy class.

You can sign up for painting, guitar drawing, photography cooking, or language dancing classes in your community college.

Stay clear of Drugs and Alcohol

I'm not here today to tell you why alcohol and other drugs are harmful to your health. It's not right for me to make that claim. However, I will say that they will only prolong the discomfort that you are likely be forced to confront.

You will not be able to overcome the trauma of this breakup simply by drinking and taking substances. Although you may feel temporarily better after smoking a joint or sipping a few beers however, it is certain to get worse after the effects have worn off. The pain will be much worse, often for days following.

Avoid using drugs to mask your hurt. If your friends are trying to pressure you to stop, simply state that you're abstaining from alcohol consumption or taking substances. If they want to know what the reason is, tell them you're doing it for reasons of health. If your friends are unable to grasp why you don't want to be a jerk and then perhaps you need to think about the amount of time you've spent with that person.

Strength Building Tool

I would like you to begin taking note of your negative thoughts toward yourself when they arise. Through the day, be aware of yourself when you think things that are negative about you This could be, for instance:

* I'm extremely messy. Why can't keep my home clean.

* I am obese and slack.

* Nobody will ever be able to love me, and I'm not worth anything.

* My ex-wife resented me due to the fact that I was an uncontrollable loser.

* I'm unable to accomplish anything correctly.

"My manager is about to make me redundant because I'm not able to concentrate at work.

* I'll never meet anyone who is as great as my former.

The life I have lived is an complete failure.

* I'm hopeless.

Each time you are confronted in one of these situations or other negative thoughts about yourself(negative thoughts about other people or objects are not part of this exercise) I would like you to say "CANCEL" out loud. After that, I would like you to say an easy compliment loudly and the less tinier the better.

* I was dressed very good today!

* The lamb that I grilled cooked at dinner the other night was amazing!

* I delivered an incredible talk at work today!

See how I decorated my bedroom!

* I just performed the Beatles" track perfectly on my guitar!

* I am very proud of myself for waking up early this morning.

If you're in public, or in the presence of other people, and can't say this loudly (nor would you) simply say "cancel and breathe quietly and then come up with an appropriate compliment to yourself inside your head.

Don't be surprised if notice yourself slipping into negative thinking constantly! Your upbringing, childhood and bad parenting have instilled negative patterns of thinking that are low in self-esteem into your. It's likely that you've been practicing ways to make yourself feel bad at an early age, which could be 20-40 or more than 60 years of negative thinking! We're going to change this one time and permanently.

This activity can change your life. But, it won't be simple in any way. It will require constant discipline and concentration for your efforts, particularly for the first few days.

Chapter 4: Inner Therapy

Anger

We, as codependents, have been taught to shut down our anger. We were penalized for showing anger when we were young. When our parents would become angry with us and we would show any anger back We were ridiculed for it and then penalized.

If one of our parents displayed anger or anger and we were conditioned to believe that we wouldn't be like them and would do everything we could to be different from their parents. It should be no surprise that we frequently avoid anger in order to appear courteous and demonstrate that we're not our parents.

However, it is more often the case that this causes us to lash out in a sudden way when we're unable to contain it within. Perhaps you've yelled at your ex-partner for no apparent reason, but they're unaware that anger has been building up inside of you for a long time. Instead of releasing everything in one go and letting it all out in a constructive, healthy way, you end up sealing it away until you're unable to keep it inside.

Have you noticed that your behavior dramatically changes when you are with your parents? Are you frequently annoyed by everything either of them does? This is usually because of unresolved childhood anger that's residing within your.

If you are waking up in the late at night and in a state of denial to go to sleep, then you're probably experiencing unresolved anger. From now on, you're not going to be able to control or be afraid of your anger. Anger is a vital emotional response that is genetically inherited by us. If it were so damaging to us then we wouldn't evolved to experience it.

This doesn't mean I'd like you to publicly exhibit your anger, or turn into an angry person! Actually, the reverse is true. I have listed three good ways below to release your anger. After you have incorporated these techniques you'll begin to notice how much more relaxed that you are on a regular basis. You won't be compelled to occasionally express your anger, usually toward people who are not involved in it. This was a first for me!

Tool for releasing anger (The techniques are listed below in ascending order of effectiveness)

1. Bat Method

Purchase a baseball bat made of plastic at the 99 cents shop. If you don't possess a 99c shop near you, then go for an aluminum-based lightweight bat at an ordinary sporting goods store. If you're at home by yourself take your bedding off the bed's corner because we do not want you to damage the furniture or anything else. Then, raise your bat above your head using both hands and then hit your bed as hard as can, without over-exerting your body. Repeat this process until you feel that you've let go some tension. One tip to use is to consider something that your ex-partner did to you. I also thought about painful memories from my childhood. Anything that can upset you is likely to cause.

2. Screaming

If you're alone inside your vehicle, open up the windows and turn on the music loud if you are in the vicinity of other people. You can shout and scream about your ex-partner without inhibitions; scream and say whatever is in your head. Make use of the bat method to bring out anger when you're not anger enough.

3. Angry Letters

Send angry emails or letters to the person/thing that you are angry with. You can either the letter to yourself or compose an email that is addressed to yourself. Allow your thoughts to flow freely and don't worry about punctuation or grammar , there is no one who will read them other than you. I wrote numerous letters to my ex and they brought me immediate relief.

These tools may be unnatural to a lot of users. It's okay. For these tools to be efficient, you need to follow them exactly as I described earlier. For instance, don't make use of one hand instead of two when hitting your bed with a bat.

Online/Mobile Dating Apps - Stay Away

Here are the top five reasons I'm not using any mobile or online dating apps:

We live in a time of instant pleasure. We can purchase products on Amazon to have it delivered at our doorstep within two days, pay cash to one another in a matter of minutes and feel proud of our achievements when we get 100+ likes on a Facebook profile image in just only a few hours.

A hookup culture with no commitment is growing and a lot of people I know are navigating through relationships, but are still trying for someone they feel comfortable with.

You can choose what you want take from the following list. I believe that all human beings share the same needs and needs deep in our souls. We subconsciously seek the same things: love, intimacy, and connection.

1. Life is about delayed gratitude When I reflected on the times when I was satisfied with me and my direction I was taking in my own life main concept throughout the years was that I didn't look for immediate

satisfaction. I was aware that things will unfold the way they were supposed to in enough time. As a man in my 20s, I've gone through my plenty of changes and ups. But, looking for Tinder is just as harmful as drinking a glass of wine. You're desperate for someone else to love you , because you're struggling with to accept yourself.

2. To face reality We are a species, and it seems like we are moving toward an emotional insensitivity. We're not able to deal with our emotions , and always seeking out the best and avoiding lows at all cost. Tinder acts as a bandage for our souls. Growth in emotions and a genuine sense of self-worth is a result of accepting our emotions of despair, boredom and sadness. These feelings will not destroy us. They will, in fact, help us to experience negative emotions and learn from these feelings.

3. To Reach My Goals When I was using dating websites for a week, once I started to meet attractive women, I began to feel a false sense satisfaction. This immediately

decreased my determination to reach my objectives in my life. The feeling of being accepted by someone else's gender biologically triggers a feeling of insecurity. My objectives don't require me to sit to a 9-5 job or living an uninvolved lifestyle created by the mass media and large business created for us.

4. To meet the right girl My idea of a perfect partner has evolved over time. I was accustomed to following my natural instinct to seek out one who was like my Mom because I was naturally drawn to this. However, these traits do not allow me to have a healthy and happy relationship. My partner must have an assertive self-image and be able of facilitating an energizing and caring relationship. We must complement each other but not be dependent on one another.

5. To find real intimacy - Like many men of today I was once convinced that meeting each week a new woman was exciting and proved my worth to myself and other people. Refraining from commitment is a

sign that you're afraid to reveal your real persona with another. I've been there, and can look back at the times that I was consciously hindering relationships that could have flourished due to my fear of having of being vulnerable. This goes from not being at ease with the person you are within. Although I'm not looking for an individual to share my life with, I would like to find someone who I can open myself up to and develop a connection with. Tinder can certainly provide me with the person I want.

Recognition List Tool

Continue to work towards developing your strength base is a continuous process that requires constant effort. You will eventually be able to. The next tool will be a good complement to the tool for building strength in week 2.

Exercise to Recognize List

Get a piece of lined paper. At the top, write "List Recognization". Below, on the next line write exactly: "These are things I believe I am doing well".

The objective is to list 10 to 15 things you can do better in this checklist. The less trivial the list, the more beneficial. For example, my list was comprised of:

* I do a great job of keeping my hair on my face.

* I cook amazing tacos with chicken shredded. I'm a fantastic cook.

My self-control is robust.

* I'm very efficient at organizing my room.

It is recommended to go through this list two times each day. I would recommend first reading it upon waking up and then before going to sleep. When you are reading it at one of these times you will read it aloud. You don't have to worry about it, you can whisper in case you're afraid people will hear you!

Chapter 5: What Is Borderline Personality Disorder?

This part is intended to provide you with an unmistakable real-world image of BPD. In the event that you suspect that you or someone near you might have BPD It is important to know exactly what it means.

Before you get started on this article, it's crucial to be aware that you aren't able to determine to be suffering from BPD. Despite the fact that you might learn about some of the side effects associated with BPD and even believe "That it's me!" You should consult with an specialist (an analyst, specialist, or a specialist who studies mental disorders) determine if you truly are suffering from BPD.

The process of determining whether you be suffering from a mental disorder is like trying to determine if you be suffering from malignant growth or coronary disease. It is best to consult with an expert make the determination since you do not have the tools and abilities or viewpoint needed to draw the right decision.

In the event you make an error in your diagnosis and you don't receive the proper help. I've met some people who believed they were suffering from BPD but ended up with another disorder that was like bipolar confusion and posttraumatic stress disorders.

Also, because the medicines prescribed for malignant growth may not be identical to those prescribed for coronary disease, every emotional or mental disorder needs the use of a different treatment. So, you'll need to make sure that your conclusions are accurate the best method to achieve this is to talk to a professional. In this regard, you can use this section to learn more about the nature of BPD is all about and to demonstrate signs of improvement in understanding of the negative effects that accompany this condition.

MENTAL DISORDERS, PERSONALITY DISORDERS and BPD

An individual with a personality disorder an authentic way of identifying with the world around us that isn't working well at all. Additionally, these disorders can create extreme pain and create difficulties seeing someone else or cause disorders to arrive at goals in everyday life, (for example, objectives that include pursuing or keeping an ideal job). There are many different kinds of personality disorders that include avoidant, fanatical, anxious, insecure, jumpy and schizotypal dramatic, narcissistic, standoffish and, of course Borderline personality disorders. A personality disorder typically is a sign of having several issues that have been affecting you for some time.

Most of the time it is necessary to be an adult to be able to determine if you be a sufferer of an emotional disorder. Whatever the case, people found to be suffering from an emotional disorder as adults typically claim to suffered from these issues for any length of time they can remember. Therefore, we can recognize that a lot of people were affected by these disorders when they were young.

Being diagnosed with a personality disorder doesn't necessarily mean you are a flawed person or that you have a poor personality or are an unpleasant or unlikable person. The assumption is that those who suffer from personality disorders have certain aspects of their personality that causes problems for them as well as other people. However, we do not believe this, due to two reasons.

The second reason is that this phrase suggests that the issue is in your own mind and that even if there was a chance that you can fix it yourself , everything would be normal. It is hard to argue with this viewpoint as well. There's a lot of evidence to suggest that the environment (for instance injuries, stress or misuse and many other causes) plays a significant role in a variety of mental disorders, such as personality disorders. Additionally, putting the disorder in you could cause shame and negative reactions in relation to other people.

Finally the term "personality disorder" is also a recommendation that, when you suffer from an emotional disorder, you've consistently been affected by it (its component that makes up your character, a part of what defines you as the person the person you're) and generally be suffering from it. As you'll see in Part 4, in every instance, there's proof that BPD isn't the only case to persist as people might think that it might. As such being diagnosed with BPD does not mean that you are a flawed person or that you'll constantly battle the disorder that you're suffering from at this moment.

It is merely a way of saying that you've got an instance of thinking, feeling, and even behavior that may hinder your ability to live a full and satisfying of living, hold your connections securely or reach your goals. The issue is the DSM-IV relies in the event that a mental disorders are an array of illnesses or clinical conditions. The DSM-IV uses the concept of an "infection model" to describe mental disorders that connect them to an illness (brokenness) in the individual (or within the environment) similar to what it is the case have a diabetes diagnosis, pneumonia or other similar illnesses. The issue with this model is that mental illness doesn't look like the diseases do. First of all it isn't possible to "get" mental illness as you would contract pneumonia. In addition, unlike illnesses like the mental disorder has been found to be unrelated to any physical disorder which could cause them. Thirdly, many of the negative effects that accompany the disorder that is explicit (for instance and in the case of wretchedness) are also present in various diseases, so the distinction between these disorders is unclear. It is evident to physicians that an individual suffers from diabetes and the malignant bosom. Fourthly, consider the things you think, do or feel.

The assumption is that certain things you perform, think or feel could indicate the presence of a disorder that is hidden. That's a big leap to make. Researchers aren't able to look inside someone's cerebrum or body to find an underlying disorder, like they would when they locate an autocinogenic tumor. Fifthly, the illness model, like people with personality disorders causes the disorder for majority of you. In the following illustration, should you suffer from BPD there is a substantial proportion of the conditions you struggle with are associated with conditions that exist on earth in contrast to the illnesses that you have. In addition, the changes you'll need to take to feel more content could be altering your nature or your behavior, thinking or feel. So, we acknowledge that the things you think, do and feel is far more significant than if you are confused.

BPD'S HISTORY BPD

The general consensus is that there are two major types of disorders and mental illness. The first, known as despondency was comprised of patients who were aware about the real world but they suffered from a passion disorder such as the nervousness or sadness disorder.

Psychosis was a different classification was for patients with unusual thoughts and experiences, (for instance, visualisations) which were not categorized in a typical way or even a general rule. These patients were found to have been an overly cluttered, for instance, schizophrenia. Patients who didn't suffer from problems that were sufficiently real to warrant being classified as insane (as the reasoning and experiences were not located in reality) However, those who were too troubled to even be considered masochists. classified as borderline.

Therapists employed the term "fringe" for patients who had painful memories, observing both the wonderful and the terrible traits of individuals at the same time that led chaotic and anxious lives and who were often truly distressed. The majority of these views concerning BPD resulted from the experiences of a certain group of patients and did not rely on research that was logical. Since the beginning of time doctors have conducted numerous tests. Results from these exams have identified a myriad of important characteristics which are the basis of what we call borderline personality disorder which includes issues with controlling emotions, inappropriate behavior as well as relationships and personality disorders.

The people who suffer from BPD will never be considered to be in the realm of psychosis and anxiety. The science is helping us maintain the beliefs about BPD that seem to be true and get rid of the outdated notions about BPD which don't seem to be precise.

THE TYPES AND FEATURES BORDERLINE PERSONALITY DISEASE

BPD is a tumultuous state of anxiety and disordered emotions. People with BPD are insecure about their emotions, their thinking as well as their relationships, character, and behavior. People who suffer from BPD are prone to rough relationships and are frequently afraid of being abandoned. On the inside, people who suffer from BPD think they're riding a rollercoaster, and their feelings bouncing everywhere and everywhere.

They might also have difficulty dealing with outrage (either experiencing outrage outbursts or becoming so scared of anger that they keep an appropriate distance from It). The people who suffer from BPD behave recklessly (they are quick to act without a sense) when they are stressed decide to commit suicide or engage in self-harm. In most cases, those suffering from BPD have difficulty understanding of who they are and, as a result, they are here and there are unable to think clearly and remaining calm when they're stressed.

The most effective treatment for BPD is:
Feeling DYSREGULATION

It is a reference to feelings of insecurity (counting rapid state of mind changes) and difficulties in regulating emotions. The people who suffer from BPD struggle with their feelings and are often overwhelmed by their feelings. In reality there are a few experts who have stated that feeling dysregulation is the primary condition for people with BPD. However, only a handful of people believe that the vast majority of issues that those who suffer from BPD struggle with come from feeling dysregulation. Mental and emotional resentments and difficulty controlling resentment are two symptoms that are a result of BPD that fall within this category.

MOODS AND TEMPERAMENTAL EMOTIONS

People with BPD frequently react to situations which aren't likely to affect other people as strongly. For instance, in the chance you are suffering from BPD it is possible that you are extremely angry about something that someone else's behavior or state or say, or you might notice that you worry more efficiently than other people. Just a simple or a different look could suffice to send you into a tizzy spiral. Because people who suffer from BPD respond in a genuine way to many things, they frequently discover that their emotions can be an exhilarating trip. They could be joyful in one moment, then unhappy or angry the next moment.

Extreme Anger or a tenseness in controlling Anger

INTENSE anger or difficulty controlling ANGER IS A PARTICULAR Feature of BPD.

Individuals suffering from BPD could be extremely agitated or angry by certain things that aren't likely to cause a stir in other people.

It is also possible that they are not in control when they explode, throwing things and yelling at people or being consumed by anger that they don't know how to handle it. Despite the fact that anger is a symptom of BPD however, we've observed when working with people with BPD that feelings of shame, pity and blame tend to be much more grounded and difficult to accept. Some people who have BPD seem to spend more energy in being angry with themselves than any other individual.

RELATIONAL RELATED

The term "relational dysregulation" refers to having difficulty when it comes to relationships with others. This doesn't mean that you're a bad or insignificant person. In reality, those who suffer from BPD are often very captivating at drawing people in, captivating and fragile. In the end the way, they'll generally fight with their relationships in two fundamental ways such as temperamental connections, and the fear of surrender.

Intense and SPECIAL RELATIONSHIPS

Individuals suffering from BPD frequently are prone to "rough" connection that can be insane and riotous. Indeed, their ferocious energy and vigor causes them to be unable to manage their connections. If you are lucky enough that you suffer from BPD it is possible that sometimes things go extremely for your connections, but at other times it seems that everything is self-destructing. You may be happy with joy, in awe, and elated for a moment, but next minute, you could be irritated and discontented and have a negative view of your relationships.

The main idea connects, comparable to emotions, can be an exciting journey, and they can swiftly go from being wonderful and depressing. If you suffer from BPD Your connections could be a source of contention or battles. You may also experience physical or mental abuse.

CONDUCT DYSREGULATION

Conduct dysregulation means that your behavior is erratic (and potentially dangerous or harmful) and has a negative impact on your daily life. People with BPD often battle the disorder in two main ways: reckless hasty behavior and self-harm.

SELL AND IDENTITY DISREGULATION

When there is a problem with self- and personality regulation the person doesn't have a stable or reasonable perception of who the person is. The person in question may be unable to feel complete a large period of time.

SUBJECTIVE DYSREGULATION

When there is a the disorder of subjective dysregulation, a person is prone to negative thinking, and an inability to connect with self or reality when one is stressed. It is important to remember this that these kinds of disorders aren't usually found and are typically experienced when people with BPD have a large quantity of pressure or are very troubled.

SPOILER-INVOLVED THOUGHTS, DISSOCI

experiencing stress

One disorder is now considered to be suspect or negative or "distrustful" thinking about other people's intentions. In the event that you are suffering from this condition, it doesn't suggest that you're naive or crazy. It could be that you're schizophrenic or even insane. This means that when you worry, you become worried or concerned about what others think of your appearance. It is possible to begin to accept that others are trying to be cruel to you, abuse you or cause trouble everywhere.

It is also possible to think that people take a look at you, and are thinking of negative or critical thoughts regarding you (for instance, "He's fat," "She's infuriating," "I don't care about the way she looks"). These kinds of encounters typically occur when you're under stress or you are upset but they aren't happening often when things are going smoothly. Another component of psychological dysfunction is the feeling of separation. Separation is the feeling of being watched and scattered with a hazy mental state and not being aware of your surroundings or feeling like you're not in your body.

Certain people experience feelings of floating to the top of the world and looking down at their bodies as well as the people who are around them. In the event that they are in BPD the separation occurs when under stress. Separation is a great strategy to escape troubles. If you are in the unlikely event that your boss dismisses you and you are nervous, agitated and angry You can contemplate the situation the situation in a lucid way for a few minutes in order to get rid of the stress or anxiety.

The problem with separation in the first place is that it doesn't reveal everything, and you can perform actions while segregating that can be risky (for instance, suicide attempts) or things you don't remember for a while (for instance, a risky single-night rendezvous).

How do you determine If you are suffering from BPD?

We have discussed it earlier, the best method to determine whether you are suffering from BPD is to talk with a specialist who can an analysis. Different kinds of experts in psychological wellbeing create analyzes, such as experts and clinicians. Therapists are medical specialists who have particular training in prescription-based and mental medications.

Analysts and therapists typically find themselves in a position to conduct an extensive analysis and come to the decision. Some of the people who make findings include social laborers, people with master's degrees in brain science, or who have master's degrees in the field of the field of brain science.

We recommend that you search for an expert who is experienced in the field of experience in preparing and involvement with personality disorders and receive a thorough examination. Because BPD is a long-running way of being a part of other people in the same way (and is a condition that many people have struggled with for the entirety of their lives) It is possible that finding out if you have BPD can take a bit of time.

Despite the fact that it is difficult to tolerate when you want to know what's going on with you, a significant decision is vital and may need a few plans and a lot of conversation. It's also important that the professional you work with is able to distinguish BPD from various other signs that could be a sign of BPD such as major sadness or bipolar disturbance.

Chapter 6: Signs Of Borderline Personality Disorder

People suffering from BPD have a wide range of mood swings, and can be prone to instability and anxiety. Borderline Personality Disorder influences your self-esteem as well as how you interact with other people, as well as the way people treat you. It is not common for everyone to experience the disorder.

Borderline Personality Disorder (BPD) sufferers may suffer from mood swings and doubts about their perception of themselves and their place on the planet.

The people with Borderline personality disorder like to watch things repeatedly just like everything good or bad things. People's views on them are subject to change. A person who is seen as a friend on one occasion could be viewed as an enemy one day, or even an intruder.

The fluctuating emotions can result in an unstable and tense relationship. Some individuals experience just a handful of symptoms, whereas others exhibit a multitude of symptoms. These symptoms are often triggered through seemingly regular events. For example, those suffering from borderline personality disorder might be angry and unhappy at the slightest interruption from the people they consider close for example, when they travel on business journeys.

The intensity or frequency, their age and the length of time they can are expected to last. In accordance with the Diagnostic and Statistical Manual Diagnostic Framework, some of the most prominent symptoms and signs may include:

The efforts of family and friends to keep from abandoning their real or imagined.

Personal relationships that are unstable and fluctuate between different ideologies like;

"I'm completely in love!"

"I hate it"

Anger and rage-filled feelings that last for a long time or emptyness.

Inappropriate, extreme or out of control anger that is uncontrollable, severe or inappropriate .This is often coupled with guilt and shame.

Unrealistic Feelings that you are disconnected from your own thoughts , thoughts of identity, or "out of the body" feelings of stress and anxiety due to stress. Extreme stress episodes can trigger brief psychological episodes.

Doing everything to avoid extreme fear of departure whether it is real or imagined rejection or separation.

Rapid changes in self-identity as well as self-image which require changing your goals and values and making you feel guilty or feel as if you don't really exist.

Paranoia that is triggered by stress and interaction with the world, ranging from just a few minutes up to several hours

Protecting your achievement by influencing and addressing dangerous behaviors, like gambling reckless driving or sex that is unsafe and spousal relationships and binge eating usage, or even abandoning a job that is good or ending a relationship that is positive.

In response to the risks of suicide, or fears of being judged or injured, people are often isolated or disregarded.

The duration of the intense mode ranges between a few hours and several days. It could include extreme emotions like anger, joy embarrassedness, anxiety, or embarrassment.

The constant feeling of emptyness

Anger that is extreme, inappropriate like a constant losing temper bitterness, sarcasm, or physical violence.

The attempt to not give up on real or imaginary for example, starting the process of forming an intimate (physical or emotionally) relationship or attempting to cut off contact with the person you love

Some of the most dangerous and shocking behaviors that include having a bad time and having sex that is not secured or drug abuse, reckless driving and eating food. If the behavior is prevalent in high moods or during an high energy state, it could be an indication of a problem, but not an alteration of the norm.

Suicidal thoughts frequently reoccur or threats

Mode that is extremely variable and severe that can last between a couple of hours and several days

The constant feeling of being empty

Inappropriate, intense anger or difficulty controlling anger

It is difficult to trust, and this is often accompanied by an an irrational fear for other people's intentions

Feelings of personalization Feelings of customization, for example, feeling disconnected from yourself, the feeling of seeing yourself outside of your body or feeling like you're being unreal

Symptoms Explained

In the hope that people might abandon their loved ones. This is why they may leave those who cannot leave others - in situations where others do not feel the same or take it as a personal attack.

Borderline personality Disorder is defined by an emotional disorder. This is the presence of a constant, immediate emotional and traumatizing emotional state that is not under any control for the person suffering from it. The disorder makes it difficult for people with problems to establish and keep relationships. They also have difficulties controlling their disorderly and reckless behavior. They often have a tendency to come up with their own ideas of what they're like.

People with borderline personality disorder usually have long-running relationships that begin and abruptly end. The reason for this can be caused by two factors:

The fear of being abandoned

Their propensity to quickly scold and then criticize others individuals

For the first time, when a student was not willing an opportunity to socialize the girl was frightened and was hurt. He suddenly realized that his acquaintance was leaving him, and assaulted one of his classmates, beat him, and claimed that his friend had left him. It was clear that the other student broke off the friendship.

For people with the disorder known as borderline personality, these events are frequent and can become overwhelming. Extreme emotions like anxiety, fear, distress as well as sadness, anger, and embarrassment could last for a couple of hours, and can last for several days.

When people are overwhelmed and angry people with borderline personality disorder are also hesitant. People may engage in actions like cutting their legs and arms as well as other suicide-related actions. Individuals may engage in the followingways:

Drunks and Alcohol in excess

Shopping that they aren't able to be able to

Gamble excessively

Not eating well and developing unhealthy eating habits

Cleaning and Benching

In the most difficult situations people may attempt to commit suicide or even think about suicide in depth. The majority of people who are involved in this kind of problem are constantly evaluating their relationships to see if they are in trouble and anticipate being abandoned by others.

They seek to put them, their friends and other things into "all excellent" and "all bad" categories without any middle line between them.

These are the reasons why minor issues could lead to the ending of the relationship. However, regardless of how fast the relationship is over the majority of people with borderline personality disorder actually are fearful of loneliness because they believe they're not able to deal with the issues themselves. Borderline personality disorder during combat is often exhausting and a source of anxiety.

The people who suffer from this condition suffer from intense psychological, emotional, and physical discomfort constantly. They're not even sure what they're really like. In one moment, someone might think that he is an ideal person, but in the next moment, they will view themselves as poor and unworthy. People's opinions about them change quickly. The person is eager to believe in others, however, simultaneously, does not believe that other people are reliable. This confusion could cause a person to feel:

Empty

Sad

Hollow

In addition to the heightened disturbances individuals suffering from borderline personality disorder may feel as if they've left their bodies during times of anxiety and forget the events that took place. The aforementioned periods of isolation just increase the anxiety of self. In addition, and even more disturbing it is possible to experience a period of deceit which can happen when there is depression or stress. Relationships that are unusually turbulent or unstable (such as being someone else's idealand and then resenting them in a severe way). Feeling unsure about yourself and not having a clear idea of who they are, or what you should think about your own self. It could be dangerous (e.g. cash before spending money reckless sexual activity or use of harmful alcohol or drugs reckless driving, having bananas) or acting inappropriately.

Self-harming, suicide, or even thinking and talking about suicide. Feeling short-lived but extreme emotional 'low', an anxiety or irritability. It is typically only just a few hours at a time but it could be longer. It is a constant feeling of being empty inside.

Experimenting with anger that is intensely extreme, and proportional to the cause of anger and then being unable to manage it (such as feeling depressed or fighting). In times of stress, people may feel a sense of doubt or sensations of being disconnected from their body, emotions or environment. There are several symptoms to be understood associated with Borderline Personality Disorder which are listed below:

The fear of losing hope

Relationships that are unstable

Blurring or altering your image

Poor Self-treating

Self-Harming

High Emotional Swings

Feelings of emptyness and constant sadness

Explosive Temper

Inexplicably or out of sync with the reality

The fear of losing hope

People suffering from BPD frequently feel lonely or lonely. Even something that is unpleasant, such like a loved one being home late , or taking an extended weekend, can cause extreme worry. It could be a desperate attempt to keep the person near.

You could make a beeline, kiss, begin fighting or track your girlfriend's movements or physically block the person from going away. However, this can have an opposite effect on others who send people away.

Relationship that is not stable

The people with BPD experience relationships that can be traumatic and also short-lived. It is possible that you will soon fall in love, thinking that every person you meet can bring you happiness but then be disappointed.

Your relationships appear perfect or fantastic, but there is no middle line. Your friends, loved ones or family members might think that they are becoming emotionally affected due to your shifting from perfect to disapproval and anger.

Blurring or altering your image

If you suffer from BPD the way you feel can be erratic. Sometimes , you may feel positive about yourself, and at other times, you feel like you're a jerk or think you are as a bad person.

You could spend money you don't have and eat, speed, drive recklessly or shoplift, perform risky sexual activities or abuse of alcohol or drugs. These risky behaviors may help you feel more relaxed in moments, however they can be detrimental to yourself and the people in your vicinity.

Self-Harming

Self-harming behaviour that may also include suicide threats or attempts to commit suicide. It is normal for those who suffer from BPD to commit suicide and intentional self-harm. Suicidal behavior includes thoughts of suicide, making threats or threats to commit suicide, or even attempting suicide.

Self-harm includes all attempts to harm yourself with no intention of taking your own life. The most common types of self-harm are burning and biting.

Extremely emotional Swings

The mood swings and feelings that are unstable are typical of BPD. At times you may feel excitement, and then, the nextmoment, you feel the anger. Small things that people do not notice could send you into a tailspin of emotions.

These mood swings can be quite extreme, yet they go disappear quickly (unlike the mood swings associated with bipolar disorder or depression) generally lasting only several minutes or hours.

Feelings of emptyness and constant sadness

People suffering from BPD often speak of feeling empty like there is an empty space or vacuum within the person. The feeling of being unfulfilled is overwhelming which is why you might seek to fill in the gap by eating, drugs or sexual stimulation. However, nothing really fills you up.

People suffering from BPD frequently struggle with skeptical thoughts or misguided beliefs about the role of others. Under pressure it is possible to become disconnected from reality. It's possible to feel hazy or distant, or even feeling like you're outside of your body.

Chapter 7: Utilizing Mindfulness To Manage Emotions

Resolving narcissistic abuse can be one of the most challenging things you'll ever have to face. It requires lots of work to discover the motivation to overcome the pain that has taken over your life, to a more positive future. The most normal response to abuse is to feel the feeling of pain. The life you have lived is broken and your heart breaks and you are devastated. But it's not over. There are solutions available for you Effective solutions that will aid you in getting the life you want.

Meditation

Narcissistic abuse causes victims to experience emotional turmoil. The type of trauma that you endure from a relationship like this can have lasting consequences in your daily life. A highly effective methods to heal, manage and conquering the negativity you encounter from a narcissist, is to practice meditation. Meditation can be beneficial for almost any illness that can be duc to stress or is exacerbated by it. Meditation can help your body relax, and in the process decreasing your metabolism rate, increasing the heart rate and lowering blood pressure (Huntington 2015). It also aids in making sure the brain to function correctly and also helps you breathe more easily. Once you've learned to relax by meditation, tension in your muscles will release out of your body and away from your muscles , where tension is abounds.

The greatest benefit of meditation is that you are able to practice it even if you are working a full schedule. It only takes only a few minutes a day and you'll be well on the journey to recovery. When you meditate, make sure to be mindful of your breathing. Take note of the air that is flowing into and out of your body. This can help you focus by following the route that the air flows into and out of your body. It's among the most efficient ways to get calm.

As the air moves into or out of you, you should examine your body to pinpoint those areas where tension is at its highest.

Be aware of your thoughts to ensure that you know what you're trying to overcome by meditative practice. It's okay to experience the overwhelming feelings however, do not be judging yourself. Recovery isn't a sprint. It could take just a few times however, your determination will get you through.

Don't be afraid of your feelings. Your emotions are an integral part of the person you are. It's normal to react in a specific way to someone's actions and behaviour toward you. Accept the emotions and get rid of the negative feelings. Meditation can help make the neural pathways that connect to or from your brain stronger and healthier by increasing the density in grey matter. It helps you become mindful of your emotions and feelings over time, and as you progress you can break the harmful relationship you shared with your victim of narcissism.

Stress and trauma can affect the brain, causing disruption to brain regions that control memory, planning as well as learning, focus and even emotional balance. Through time the practice of meditation has proven to be an effective method to overcome these difficulties by improving the performance of the amygdala, the hippocampus and the prefrontal cortex.

If you are an abuser who is narcissistic Once your abuser gains the upper hand in your life, you are left with only one option: follow the instructions of their abuser. Meditation can help you get into control again. It allows you to take back your life and heal, and be empowered to conquer any challenges that you faced under their control.

Group therapy

Group therapy is among the options to consider in the process of healing from narcissistic abuse. The first thing you'll learn during groups is the fact that it is not possible to cure the abusive narcissist. What you will discover is how to manage the narcissism.

The majority of people are urged to get out of toxic relationships because they are only hurts and suffering from them. Narcissists are relentless in their search for love satisfaction, attention and attention. They know that what they want is not possible to attain, but they believe in believing that they can help their goals come true.

Therapy for those who have been abused by a narcissist beneficial because it gives you something you haven't experienced for quite a while the assistance. Every time it is revealed the stories of other members of the group and you realize that you're not the only one. The overwhelming emotions you've been experiencing become less overwhelming as you realize that there are others in the world who can relate to the things that have been going through your mind.

Although group therapy does have its advantages, you'll need to take part in order to benefit from these advantages. The willingness to heal indicated in the way that you're taking the first step in your journey to seek assistance. Be committed to your therapy sessions by making the pledge of what you'd like to get from it. After you've signed up the process, be involved. It may not be straightforward at first as you must open up to strangers but you will soon get used to it. It's fine to be quiet and listen to people talk about their experiences initially. Once you feel at ease opening up, you can share your story. Be aware that it becomes easier with time as you continue to share. Never hold back. Therapy is a secure space. When you share your story it's not just sharing with the group your suffering, but you may help another person in the group talk about their own experiences.

Cognitive behavioral therapy

Cognitive behavior therapy (CBT) is an effective therapy that blends both behavioral and cognitive therapy to help people overcome traumatizing events that took the power away from them. Cognitive therapy concentrates on the effect your beliefs and your thoughts play in your life. Likewise, it is about finding and changing harmful behavior habits (Triscari and colleagues 2015)

CBT works because the therapist doesn't simply sit and listen, they also serve as your personal coach. It's a healthy and healthy interaction where you can learn effective strategies that will assist you in managing your life more effectively. It helps you recognize your emotional reactions, behavior and thoughts.

CBT is an ideal treatment for victims of narcissistic assault because it aids them in understanding the emotional impact of their experiences, spot behaviors that are problematic, in particular tendencies, and learn to manage the most challenging circumstances in their lives.

Cognitive processing therapy

CPT is an aspect of CBT. It is among the most highly recommended methods of dealing with trauma victims. Narcissistic abuse victims typically suffer a great deal of emotional trauma and may be diagnosed with PTSD. If you suffer from PTSD and experience PTSD, you may be able to perceive the world around you and the those you meet. PTSD can alter your perception of your life in these areas:

* Safety

Following an experience of the trauma of abuse, you're conditioned to feel unsafe around your self and those around you. Trauma can intensify these worries regarding security. It is a fear that you will not be able to take care of yourself and anyone else.

* Trust

Narcissists tear you until you're sunk to earth. They ensure that you not trust anyone, or even yourself. After the incident, PTSD can cause you to doubt your ability to make the right decision.

* Control

It's not enough to lose control of your life; you trust your abuser to help you navigate your way through life. Narcissism is the cause. Narcissists feel happy when they are in control of your life since they know they are in your thoughts and are able to do whatever they want with you. After leaving a narcissist PTSD can intensify a

sense of being out of control, making getting back to your feet difficult and slow.
* Esteem
One of the worst things dealing with a narcissist's behavior is how they can erode your confidence. Even the most confident individuals who have ever lived were being unable to identify who they really are or the purpose of their lives in the present. You avoid situations that require confidence and savvy decision-making, something you could have readily accepted before. Your self-image is that you are a flawed and unworthy individual.
* Intimacy
Alongside other tricks that the narcissists employ, triangulation causes you feel so unsure regarding yourself and your intimacy. It makes you feel uneasy since no one can understand your feelings, but simultaneously you don't understand why they behave in the way they do. In the aftermath of narcissistic abuse PTSD can trigger a series of flashbacks to times that your relationships were insecure. It could

cause you to have difficulty starting new relationships.

These thoughts result in negative emotions obscuring your life, such as anger, guilt depression, fear, and anger. Through CPT you will learn valuable techniques to challenge these negative emotions. Negative emotions can create an illusion of self-worth that is embedded into your mind and makes you feel like an inferior being. CPT can help you improve your self-image and the world surrounding you. It helps you overcome the negativity and gain an improved, positive and healthier perspective on your life.

Yoga

For those who have suffered trauma yoga may provide the possibility of healing. Yoga's restorative qualities are well-known to Eastern traditional societies to promote wellness. Yoga assists in establishing connections between your mind and body. It aids in staying grounded. This is among the most important things to survive a narcissistic relationship.

Yoga has been shown by the experts in past studies to be beneficial for treating various mental and physical conditions such as trauma-related issues, anxiety (Criswell, Wheeler, & Partlow Lauttamus (2014)). By combining breathing exerciseswith yoga's physical movements as well as relaxation techniques, it assists to improve your mindfulness and make you more aware of the world around you both internal and external.

The breaking up and getting out of a relationship an narcissist is only the beginning. The process of healing requires more steps. You must find your feet. It is time to put an end to your confusion, which has consumed your life until you don't have a sense of identity.

In yoga, you be focusing in breathing exercise. Breathing is among the most effective and affordable ways to get relief. If you're going through an emotional turmoil, or experiencing anxiety All you need to do is breath.

When you are feeling an urge to invite the narcissist into your life, you should find an area in which you can unwind and unwind. Relax your eyes and breathe. Concentrate on your breathing and count your breaths, and take your mind off of the issue. Yoga classes with gentle movements can assist in this regard.

Art therapy

Art therapy was developed around the belief that mental health as well as recovery can be enhanced by expressing creativity. Art therapy is not only an art form, but it is also a method which can improve mental well-being. The art therapy method has been used in psychotherapy for many years. The art therapy method allows patients to express their feelings without needing to talk to someone about their feelings.

It's a great option for people who are struggling to communicate in a way that is clear and concise. Art therapy can help you understand how to better communicate with others, reduce stress , and gain insight into your personality. By using art in therapy professionals believe that their clients can discover ways to resolve issues, deal with conflicts, relieve anxiety, develop good habits enhance or develop the interpersonal abilities of others, as well as boost their self-esteem and understanding (Lusebrink, n.d.)

Therapists who work with art have lots of tools available which can assist you in overcoming the pain of an unhealthy relationship. From collages to painting and sculpture it is all there to explore. Art therapy is suggested for those who have suffered emotional trauma and anxiety, depression and domestic abuse, as well as physical violence, or other psychological issues that result due to an abusive relationship with the Narcissist.

The distinction between the arts therapy class and an art session is the fact that with therapy the focus is on your personal experiences. Your thoughts, feelings and thoughts are important. These are the things that your narcissist friend may have forced you to give up. You'll learn amazing artistic skills and techniques but, before doing this your therapist will help the expression of your feelings from the deep inside. Instead of being focused on what you observe physically, you are taught to create objects that you can imagine or feel.

EMDR

Eye Movement Desensitization Reprocessing (EMDR) can be a different option to get rid of narcissistic abuse. This technique aids in the rewiring of your brain to be free of trauma so that it is able to process memories. Trauma exposure can cause your brain to form an underlying pattern that perpetuates the trauma you've experienced for a long period of time (Mosquera and Knipe, 2015)

Traumatic memories can cause sufferers suffering from psychological stress. EMDR is a distinct method of treatment since you don't need to discuss your feelings and issues. Instead, your brain is stimulated to alter the way that you feel for months,, or years later after you have walked away from a manipulative person.

EMDR is effective because eye movements allow the brain to relax which makes it possible to access your past memories in a way that the brain can process in a secure setting other that the one that your trauma perpetuated. After accessing your memories they can be replaced with powerful emotions and thoughts and, over time, you can let go of the trauma and begin to respond more positively to triggers that are within your surroundings. The nightmares, flashbacks, and anxieties soon fade away memories as you start to live your new life and liberate your mind from their grip.

If you are a victim of narcissistic violence Your brain is able to recall painful memories of sexual, verbal emotional, psychological, and physical violence. When you attend an EMDR therapy session, it is suggested that you focus on the specifics of traumatizing events, while simultaneously looking at other things for a brief duration.

It is what happens as you are focusing on both negative and the new positive affirmation, the memory you are experiencing is different. It is also possible to learn techniques for self-soothing to aid in separating yourself from the hurt. EMDR can help you break free of the chains that hold you back and allows your brain to think differently about the experiences you've had.

Self-hypnosis

Hypnotherapy has proven effective to assist those suffering from narcissistic abuse heal for many years. There are specific requirements which must be met to allow this therapy to be effective. You need to ensure that you are within the presence of certain factors that could trigger the process of hypnosis. Additionally, you will learn to narrow your focus and awareness. Finally let yourself freely feel your emotions without making a an intentional decision to be hypnotized.

Narcissists do not have the capacity to make real connection, instead they communicate their fears and fears of being lonely and abandoned to their victims. How do you go about getting into the trance state of hypnosis? Abuse of emotions can have a major effect on you. Hypnosis can help you unwind effortlessly.

It is a way to relax effortlessly. the things that you may not have experienced during your experience with the sexually narcissist. When you're capable of letting yourself relax without effort, you can open the doors to improving your mind and body.

Self-hypnosis is an transformative method that helps you believe in yourself and it encourages you to master important techniques for dealing with emotions that will help you overcome abuse and help you ensure your safety for the future. Every session you attend you grow stronger and more calm. The emotional turmoil you were experiencing diminish and you are more in tune with yourself and the world around you.

Self-hypnosis can also give you more clarity about the things you are living for. It helps you let go of negative thoughts and embrace peace. You're on the path of re-discovery. You see more value in yourself than ever have in your relationship with a narcissist. While you are in the sessions you are taught how to take necessary steps towards healing and progressing toward a positive direction in life. The primary thing that happens with self-hypnosis is that it makes you start anticipating the future and you believe that you can succeed in the process.

Aromatherapy

Although it may seem like you're on the end of the road and there's no way to get back there is a way to overcome an abuse of narcissism. There are many who have experienced it before, and you could achieve it as well. The process of healing from this type of trauma can be very satisfying. Every time you progress you are able to reflect on how far you've come and the progress you've made. This helps to appreciate your life and you realize how toxic it was before.

Aromatherapy is among the efforts that you are conscious of in the direction of healing and recovery from abuse by narcissists. Imagine aromatherapy in the same way as you think about exercising. If you believe you're not fit, you workout often. You could plan three or four sessions of training every week to keep you fit.

Similar to aromatherapy. Narcissists can make you in a state of emotional ill-fit. It is essential to bring your emotions into form so that you can lead a healthy and satisfying life. To get rid of stress and anxiety You must activate your amygdala. The smell of a scent is among the best methods to activate the amygdala. It is evident that there's a powerful bond between your emotions and the sense of smell. It's a connection that has existed since the age of a child.

It is believed that the sense of smell can be connected to emotional experiences regardless of whether they are positively or negatively. This is why every when you are able to smell your favourite food being cooked it brings back memories of an event you were delighted by it. It is because smells help to create comfort and also a sense of nostalgia. If the smell of a scent can transport you back to the past and help to bring back the traumas you endured through an act of narcissism.

Chapter 8: Epidemiology Factors Of Borderline Personality Disorder

The existence of intense and diverse moods, such as an impulsive anger, mania or depression that are characteristic of the disorder of borderline personality was described in the works of Hippocrates as well as Homer. The concept was revived in the latter part of the 1600s by Swiss doctor Theophile Bonet and he described the symptoms of unstable emotions , followed by unpredictability. The word "borderline" was first coined around 1938 by Adolf Stern as he described a patient group that were suffering from what he believed was mild schizophrenia, borderline neurosis and psychosis. Since the patients showed borderline signs of these disorders, the condition was referred to as"borderline..

A majority of the people who suffer with borderline personality disorder see an improvement in their condition after treatment. After long-term treatment, a number of studies found that more than

86% of those suffering with borderline personality disorder get a steady recovery. Contrary to what the majority of people believe , people with borderline personality disorder may overcome their extreme symptoms.

Epidemiology

The incidence of the disorder can be found in the range of 1%- 2percent of the overall population. Additionally, women are more likely to be affected by the disorder of borderline personality than males due to the excess of estrogen hormone. In a study from 2008 that was conducted, it was discovered that borderline personality disorder was more likely to be present at 5.6 percentage in men and 6.2 percentage for women. But, the proportion of cases that borderline personality disorder is a disorder is low according to certain experts.

This specific personality disorder is thought to cause to at least 20% of the instances of admission to psychiatric hospitals. Furthermore, this disorder contributes to 10% of all outpatient consultations for psychiatric disorders within the United States.

However the disorder known as borderline personality disorder is an extremely common disorder which has affected prisoners across the United States. The average prevalence of borderline personality disorders among prisoners in the United States is 17%. The prevalence of borderline personality disorder is high in US prisons is due to the large number of prisoners who suffer from addiction and mood disorders.

As we mentioned previously, those who suffer with borderline personality disorder may be cured of their condition. But, the process of recovery can be a shock due to the surge of emotions that flow from the sufferer. Even though this might happen, those who suffer from this disorder can continue to live normal, healthy lives. Below are some treatment and management options that are available to individuals who suffer from borderline personality disorder.

Psychotherapy Therapy is the most commonly used method of treatment for those with borderline personality disorder. Treatments usually are dependent on the specific requirements that the individual sufferer has. People suffering from borderline personality disorder must undergo long-term psychotherapy to be more successful in being able to manage their illness. There are various types of psychotherapy treatment patients are able to undergo. Below is a description of the various kinds of psychotherapy treatment options for those with this disorder.

Treatment that is based on mentalization is a form of psychodynamic therapy. It is designed specifically for patients who suffer from borderline personality disorders. The main goal of this treatment is to enhance the patient's mental health through allowing them to regain mental clarity in order to enable the psychotherapist to deal with the present psychological state that the person is in. This process is generally done as a group or individual therapy. This particular approach aims to help the patient establish a connection with their colleagues.

Transference-focused psychotherapy: This kind of psychotherapy is carried out every two weeks. It is extremely structured and specifically designed for those with borderline personality disorders. The goal of this method of psychotherapy is to lessen the self-harmful behaviour of patients.

Dialectical Behavior Therapy: This specific psychotherapy approach seeks to lower the possibility of self-harm suicidal behaviour, suicidal behaviors and addiction to drugs for people suffering from mental illness.

General psychiatric treatment Psychotherapy: This specific treatment method is a scientifically-based treatment method for the treatment of mental disorders. The treatments employed in general psychiatric treatment comprise cognitive behavioral therapy and psychoanalytic object-relation therapy.

Schema-focused therapy or schema therapy is an integrative method to treat a variety of character-logical and mental issues like the borderline disorder of personality. It blends techniques and theories like cognitive behavior therapy attachment therapy, psychoanalytic and object relations theory to treat patients.

The efficacy of psychotherapy treatments depends on the individual. But, research suggests that dialectical behavior therapy both work in treating all types that are a part of borderline disorder.

The issue when it comes to psychotherapy is it's an ongoing treatment that could create a massive financial burden on the patient as well as their immediate family. The cost of a lengthy psychotherapy session for those with borderline personality disorder is expensive. However, numerous researchers are currently making shorter versions of treatments to improve the availability of therapy to as many people as they can.

However, the expense of the therapy is not the only reason that makes this therapy difficult. Because patients with this disorder are scared of rejection psychotherapists have to be flexible in handling the negative attributes that the client may have.

Meditation

Studies have shown that meditation can result in positive changes to the brains of those who suffer from borderline personality disorder. Meditation may also provide relief of the symptoms that are characteristic of the disorder of borderline personality. Indeed, many psychiatrists suggest meditation as an therapy as an adjunct to psychotherapy.

Inpatient and Outpatient Admissions

The majority of patients suffering with borderline personality disorder have greater chance of regaining their condition when they undergo inpatient or outpatient admissions. There are a variety of facilities across the country that offer to patients who require full-time care who suffer from various mental disorders , including the disorder known as borderline personality. However, the issue with this particular management choice is that it's extremely expensive, and only a handful of people are able to afford treatment at these facilities.

What treatment is a person with borderline personality disorder select? There is no definitive solution, but it is essential to urge a person suffering from borderline personality disorder to visit a psychiatrist who can plan the best treatment plan to treat the symptoms that the person is suffering from.

Moderating Factors for Treating Borderline Personality Disorder

Similar to other forms of personality disorders There are moderating factors which can impact the efficacy of treatments for patients with borderline personality disorders. This article will discuss the various factors that affect the effectiveness of treatment and treatment for sufferers.

Executive Function

The executive function is the brain functions of individuals. It's the way we react to the various stimuli that are thrown at us. The executive functions in people with borderline personality disorder are responsible for the connection between their symptoms and the sensitivity to rejection. The symptoms are largely influenced by the cognitive functions of the brain. In other words, brain directs the person suffering from Borderline personality disorders to act in accordance with their needs and this can affect the efficacy of the treatment patients receive.

Family Environment

The immediate family environment plays a role in the development as in the healing process of a person with a disorder called borderline personality.

Self-Complexity

A person suffering from borderline personality disorder exhibits numerous traits and is prone to a range of emotions at the same time. The self-complexity of the patient makes it challenging for doctors to deal with patients suffering from borderline disorders. Patients who suffer from this condition experience an internal battle that is filled with ironies, and make it difficult for psychiatrists to help them see that they need to have a clear path for their emotional state.

Repression of thoughts

Though suppression is a typical defense mechanism used by those suffering from the disorder of borderline personality, it's an effort to avoid thinking about certain thoughts that could make vulnerable people. It makes those who suffer from borderline personality disorder more elusive and resistant to treatment.

The borderline personality disorder could be among the personality disorders easily identifiable, but it's also very difficult disorders to treat since sufferers know they have a condition however they are extremely resistant to accept changes. Yet, it's possible to treat them by a constant treatment and perseverance.

Chapter 9: Diagnostics Of The Disorder

One of the most difficult aspects of this type of disorder is determining it. The majority of people affected aren't likely to want any contact with the physician or psychiatrist who attempts to assist them, consequently, they will avoid them and refuse advice. Most of the time, it will be the family members who must see the problem and get the necessary help before the individual suffering from the disorder will receive the assistance. They won't take the initiative by themselves because they will not discover that they are suffering from any problems at all.

If you are able to get the patient with the disorder to walk through the room and be assessed, the diagnosis of this disorder is determined by the test of your clinic with a specialist in the field of mental health. The most effective way to do this is to explain the various aspects of the illness to the patient. the criteria for which are given above. Ask the patient if they feel that any of them describe them. This will make the patient more involved in the process of overcoming the disorder, making it more likely that it will work. Furthermore, a doctor is typically not going to have the time or experience working with the patient to be able to tell whether the signs are present, and offer them a generally accurate method of determining the truth about it.

If you permit the patient with this type of illness to be involved in the diagnosis, they're going be more likely to receive the support from the doctor who is going to offer them. There are some physicians who believe it's ideal to not inform their patients that they are suffering from this condition because they think that it's a source of stigma. The patient may be resistant to treatment due to having been told in the past that this is a non-treatable disease. While this is certainly a option however, there's a lot of research that shows those affected by the illness must be aware of it in order for the best treatment available.

In this examination patients are likely be asked lots of questions concerning their symptoms beginning and the severity of their symptoms. There may also be specific questions regarding how the symptoms are affecting their lives. The issues the doctor will note down include thoughts about harming others, any experiences of self-harm and all thoughts or feelings of suicide the person is having.

The diagnosis will be based on the information that the patient has reported during sessions and the things that the doctor was observed in the short amount of duration. Both of these are likely be combined to provide an accurate picture of what's going on. There are other tests that could be performed to determine the presence of borderline personality disorder present in the individual. Sometimes, some tests in the lab or physical examinations will be conducted to determine if there are any other factors which could cause the symptoms, for instance, an individual who is addicted to substances or has a thyroid issue and both can cause similar behaviors that can be observed in the borderline personality disorder.

When the problem has been identified and confirmed in a patient it's time working on giving them the care they require to remain healthy and gain their lives back to normal. While this can be a significant undertaking and may take some time however, it's essential to get it done for anyone who wants to regain their life and feel much more content. Here's more details on how the problem can be identified and one can get the help they need to feel better quickly.

International Classifications

There are several categories that you'll be able to locate which are internationally used to aid in making the diagnosis. They are useful since they permit the doctor to make the diagnosis without relying according to their personal convictions and keep things in order and consistent throughout. The concept that borderline disorder is a form of personality is a condition that has been acknowledged as such by World Health Organization

Impulsive Type

The primary type of category that is identified as the type that is impulsive. Of the factors which are listed below At minimum three needs to be present in order to identify those suffering from this kind of disorder. A tendency to be into a state of chaos or behave out. It will occur in a sudden manner and not be the result of someone else causing the problem or causing them to behave. Most of the time, the act is going take place by the individual without considering or even thinking about the possible consequences that might result from their actions. It's just something they'll perform, possibly due to a minor disagreement or some other matter which shouldn't have been any big deal but was transformed into one.

A tendency of sufferers to engage in an attitude that is deemed to be unsettling and to be in conflict with others around them. This is likely to be the case with actions which have been condemned or stopped. The person in question regularly gets in fights with those around them , and who view every little thing as a reason to get into a fight.

An issue with having powerful anger outbursts that are accompanied by anger or violence. They are not only having these issues, they lack the capacity to manage the devastation or other problems that pop up. They may appear very angry, but they'll also seem like they lack the ability to go back to calm even if they wanted.

The people who are in this situation are also likely be having a difficult time sticking to their plan of action if not able to receive immediate rewards. They might have been attracted to doing something however, in the event that it didn't bring the immediate reward they desired the most likely outcome was that they became frustrated and angry and made the decision to give up. This can occur frequently and the person will keep doing things that they know they could finish and get awarded with.

They are often moods that are unpredictable and volatile which can alter without warning. It may be challenging keeping up with these types of people.

These are the five signs that are typically encountered in those experiencing the impulsive form of the disorder. You will notice that they tend to perform actions without giving thinking about the actions they take or what will occur when they finish which could be dangerous. To be considered to have this type of disorder, they're required to have at minimum three of the issues that were mentioned earlier when they speak to their therapist at the office.

Borderline Type

The next type is the borderline. The borderline type is going to differ a bit. It takes an element from the list that was previously mentioned and add an additional item from the list which is described below. You must have minimum three of the symptoms for the type of impulsive along with the minimum of two of the below symptoms to be diagnosed with this type. A few of the signs to look out for include the following: people with this kind of personality will typically experience some confusion and discord in their self-image, as well in their personal preferences and the goals they have in their lives. They don't believe that they're worth anything and even though they desire social interaction however, they don't know why they would like to be in any way with them. They could wander around for in a state of confusion because they don't know their identity, who they really are or what they are supposed to do with their lives or what they will become of their lives. They may also be at an increased risk of getting into relationships which are typically fragile and intense. This could include the whirlwind relationships in which they get married in a matter of months however, it doesn't require to be as extreme to be a problem. Since the relationship is fragile, it's not likely to last, and because it was intense, it's likely to trigger a kind of emotional stress within the person affected by the disorder.

They are likely to put in a lot of effort to make sure they don't become lonely. They fear that they'll be awake without anyone to share their experiences or to assist them in the event of require it. The problem is compounded due to the fact that they're pushing people away and aren't very adept in recognizing other's points of viewpoint. They will do everything they can to ensure that people don't leave them on their own so that they always get the support and support they want.

They may also encounter frequent threats as well as instances of self-harm. This is typically not in the attempt to force people to behave in as they would prefer or to alter the behavior of someone else. It is more of a thing that people do in desire to get their own feelings in check. They'll struggle with their emotions, and, since they aren't in a position to keep their emotions in check it is possible that they will resort to self-harm in hopes to get some relief.

The frequent feelings they experience of emptyness. Since they don't make any plan for the future or what they would like to accomplish throughout their lifetime, they will begin be feeling empty. They don't have any objectives or long-term plans, and often will just be a wanderer about and pray that everything goes according to plan best. This could result in living a life that seems empty.

They will frequently exhibit behavior that is an impulsive. This could include things like speeding and substance abuse. The reasoning behind these actions is that it provides the sufferer with an opportunity to take a break from the negative feelings or uncontrollable emotions that they're experiencing in order to get better. The problem comes when the person starts to feel guilt-ridden about their actions and they experience a worse feeling than before.

As we've mentioned it is necessary to have several conditions that exist before one is diagnosed with this type of disorder. However, those who are in the right position should receive the assistance they require whenever they can.

Family Members

The way in which the person suffering from the disorder is treating other people close to them could be a method of diagnosing the condition. The people who suffer from this disorder will be more likely to dislike their family members and are more likely be angry with those same individuals. Most often, the person suffering from the disorder will try to distance them from their family members because they are unhappy about a minor niggle or concerned that family members will begin to notice an issue. The family members are often likely to feel insecure and annoyed by the way they relate to the person who is suffering and might be wondering how they could help make things better.

A study was conducted in 2003 that revealed that the attitudes of family members changed once they realized it was due to reasons. Most of the time the hurt and anger towards the individual suffering from the disorder would rise as family members began to realize what was happening. Although it may not appear as if it could be the case, it's often thought that these emotions are happening because families are being presented with the wrong information about the disorder . As a result, they are blamed on the person, not the actual issue.

The most effective method for family members to assist the person they cherish is to find out as much as they can about the condition. It's easy to begin reading books or watching TV shows that deal with the disorder and , while it is an excellent place to begin in certain instances but you'll find that it's usually not the right information. Find the correct and this will help you clarify the issues you're experiencing with your loved ones.

It will be equally difficult for the members of the family just as for the individual who is undergoing the situation. They are those who are emotionally hurt by their loved ones not wanting to be involved with them. It is essential that the family receive the support and therapy they need to be able to feel better about the issue. Being aware of the entire issue and how it impacts the affected family members and sufferers can help deal with the whole issue as a family.

Diagnosing Other Disorders

It is common for someone struggling with this type or disorder also to suffer from various other conditions regardless of whether they are personality disorders or another which will be present simultaneously. This makes it harder to identify the personality disorder since it could be disguised by the other symptoms. In comparison to people who suffer from any of the other personality disorders, people with borderline personality disorders will be more likely to being able to meet the criteria for other disorders, such as:

Mood disorders - this could include major depression and bipolar disorder.

Anxiety disorders: There are a variety of them that can be addressed and could comprise post-traumatic-stress disorder as well as social anxiety disorder and panic disorder.

Other personality disorders of different kinds

Substance abuse

Eating disorders, which would encompass things such as anorexia nervosa and bulimia

ADHD and Attention Deficit Hyperactivity Disorder

Somatoform disorders

Dissociative disorders

If someone with this disorder is suffering from another issue and has other issues, they shouldn't be diagnosed with the disorder until the other problem is addressed. These other issues can cause similar symptoms, and dealing with them may be a more effective approach to tackling your personality disorders. The exception is when the symptoms associated with the disorder are confirmed to have existed for several years prior to the second problem was discovered.

It is also more likely for women to be affected by one or more of the issues mentioned above, while men are likely to experience certain other issues. For instance, males tend to be more prone in terms of addiction issues, while women will suffer more eating disorders. It is crucial to take these other issues into consideration if you'd like to achieve the most effective results in managing those with borderline personality disorders. It will be virtually impossible to treat the personality disorder if you suffer from one or more of the issues mentioned above since they will cause the disorder to develop and persist even after a many sessions of therapy the course.

This is the reason that most doctors will conduct a thorough evaluation of the patient in order to find out if there is other problems evident in their patient. This makes it simpler to get rid of the personality disorder after the other issues have been addressed. This can be accomplished through a few initial therapies or by using medication to treat issues like depression and anxiety to get the most effective outcomes.

Chapter 10: Treatment And Medication

Every person's experience in the presence of such a disorder differs. Certain symptoms could be more prominent; someone else might be more agitated, while in another case, he could be more dissociative. Based on the particular circumstance and the situation the therapist will recommend the appropriate method of treatment to treat borderline personality disorders.

If someone is diagnosed with BPD it is often an overwhelming situation that makes one feel lonely because it creates stress on relationships. The people suffering from BPD require guidance from counselors to conquer this aspect of the disorder, so that they can resume their normal lives and benefit from the happiness that healthy relationships bring. Treatment for BPD can equip people with essential skills they must apply in the world to maintain social relationships. Furthermore, treatment can ease the anxiety associated with the prescribing of medications that lessen BPD symptoms.

Psychotherapy

Psychotherapy is the primary option for those suffering from mental illness, particularly those with BPD. There are many different forms that are offered in psychotherapy, all share the same goal, and that is helping patients understand how their emotions and thoughts function. It is an essential element of treatment since while medications can reduce some signs of borderline personality disorder but it can not assist patients to develop coping strategies or manage their emotions in the same way that psychotherapy does.

Psychotherapy is also vital to help people avoid taking their own lives. Therapists and other medical professionals keep in touch with the patient and keep checking their risk of suicide throughout their treatment. If a patient is suffering from extreme feelings of suicide, admission to a hospital follows.

Dialectical Behavior Therapy

The most well-known and efficient type of psychotherapy that is currently in use has been Dialectical Behavior Therapy or DBT. It was created by Marsha Linehan. It is a method of teaching people to have more control of their lives and their emotions. DBT is also a firm emphasis on emotional regulation self-knowledge, as well as the process of cognitive restructuring. DBT offers a broad method and is typically done in groups. The skills that DBT teaches is considered to be complex and not recommended for those who are struggling to grasp new concepts.

Dialectical Behavior Therapy employs two ideas: validation and dialectics. In validation, the patient is taught that their feelings are genuine, valid and legitimate. However, dialectics is a type of philosophy that teaches life should not be viewed as either black or white. It also emphasizes the necessity of accepting ideas even when they are contrary ones own beliefs.

Therapists that specialize in DBT assist those who are susceptible to suicide by guiding them through mindfulness as well as interpersonal effectiveness, emotion regulation and anxiety tolerance. When those suffering from BPD realize that there are healthier methods of dealing with and managing their emotions, the chances of self-harming and suicide are greatly reduced.

A disorder called borderline personality as other disorders of personality, can be difficult to manage. Since the aim of treatment is changing the way people view the world as well as stress and others The treatment usually takes a long time. Treatment for BPD generally lasts for at least a year long, but it can last much longer.

There are other types of psychotherapy used to treat borderline personality disorders which focus upon conflict management and the social-learning theories. These are more solutions-oriented therapies that fail to solve the primary issue of those suffering from BPD that is the difficulty in regulating their moods.

Schema Focused Therapy

Schema Focused Therapy is a form of psychotherapy whose main purpose is to pinpoint and address unhealthy ways of thinking. Certain elements of schema-focused therapy are also present within cognitive behavior therapy (CBT) and it blends it with other forms of psychotherapy.

Schema-focused therapy is based by the idea that when a person's primary childhood needs like acceptance, love and a need to be safe are not met which leads to the formation of unwholesome mental models of the world. They are known as unadaptive early schemas. They are broadly defined as patterns of thinking and behavior. They go beyond belief systems because they are deeply established patterns that impact how one thinks about and engages in interactions with other people.

The schema theory states that schemas develop when the events of one's current life are reminiscent of things that happened in the past and directly relate to the formation that schema. If someone has unhealthy schemas because of a challenging childhood, they'll eventually be prone to developing negative methods of thinking in reaction to the circumstance. Schema theory also suggests that the signs associated with borderline personality disorders typically are due to a difficult childhood in which a child might have suffered trauma, abandonment or even maltreatment from parents or both which led to the formation of schemas that are maladaptive in the beginning.

The therapy focusing on schemas for patients with borderline personality disorder aims to discover relevant schemas within an individual's life and link them to schemas that are present in previous events. The therapist helps the patient manage the emotional reactions that occur in response to the schema. They also work on addressing negative coping strategies to assist the patient in responding to the schema in a positive way. Schema-focused therapy could be a series of exercises specifically designed to stop unhealthy behavior patterns, alter the way people think and encourages the patient to express their anger.

Transference Therapy with Focus

Transference Focused Therapy uses the relationship between the patient and therapist to enhance the way the person suffering from borderline personality disorder perceives the world. Transference is the process in which emotions are transmitted from one person to the next. It is a fundamental method used in psychodynamic therapies in which it is believed that how a person is feeling about people who are important to them is passed on to their counselor. With transference, the therapy will discern what the client's interactions are with people who are in his life to assist them manage effectively relationships. In the end, the aim of the therapy focused on transference is to allow patients to enjoy maintaining relationships.

Therapists who practice transference-focused therapy believe that the symptoms of borderline personality disorders that originate from dysfunctional relationships endured in childhood persist into adulthood, and can impact the capacity of adult patients to maintain healthy, normal relationships. The interactions we experience in our relationships with the primary people we care for in the early years of our lives affect how we form self-esteem and affects the way we view the world around us. If one is not in an enjoyable connection with the caregivers in childhood, this can lead to adults not being able to connect with others and having confidence in themselves.

Research has shown that abuse or the loss of caregivers in childhood increase the likelihood of developing BPD. Because these signs have a negative consequences, and can hinder people from forming relationships with others later and affecting relationships with others, experts on BPD believe it's crucial to tackle this issue by helping people concentrate on improving their relationships with others through treatment that is focused on transference.

When it comes to this kind of therapy, there's an emphasis upon the relationships between client and the therapy. Contrary to other forms of therapy, where the therapist offers directions on what the client must do, transference-focused therapy is a method of asking the client several questions throughout the conversation as they examine their the reactions. Additionally, there is an added importance to events occurring at the moment, instead of focusing on the past. As an example instead of discussing concerns with caregivers throughout one's childhood The discussion is focused on the relationship of the client to their therapy.

Therapists who use transference-based therapy also have the ability of staying impartial, this is the main reason for why this type of therapy is so effective. They do not offer their opinions on the patients' reactions. They are also not present outside of sessions, only in emergencies.

Psychotherapy based on Mentalization

The mentalization-based treatment (MBT) is a different type of psychotherapy. It is founded on the idea that those who suffer from borderline personality disorder are having difficulty being able to think about their own thoughts. It means that people suffering from BPD cannot examine their own beliefs, thoughts or opinions, and whether they are logical and beneficial for them. A good example is that people who suffer from BPD might experience an urge to harm themselves and may end with a decision to give in, without considering the consequences that their behavior has.

MBT is important as it helps people understand that people have their own ideas and beliefs, and that your personal interpretation of their mental state may not be the most accurate. In addition, it assists people to understand that actions can have an consequences for the mindset of other people. The principal purpose in MBT is to assist people recognize their own and the mental state of others. It also helps people suffering from BPD to detach from their thoughts and determine whether they're valid. MBT is a therapy that can be found in the hospital as a type of therapy inpatient. The treatment consists of each day therapy sessions with the therapist aswell in sessions in groups.

MBT generally lasts between 18 and 18 months, but based on the requirements, patients might be required to remain an inpatient for the full length of the treatment. Certain hospitals and treatment facilities allow patients to leave at specific times throughout their treatment.

Therapeutic Communities

Therapeutic Communities (TC) are an approach to psychotherapy in which patients suffering from a variety of psychological disorders are able to interact in a controlled environment. This type of therapy is ideal for people who are struggling with emotions or who are suicidal. Through teaching them the skills necessary for healthy interactions with a variety of people, those who suffer from borderline personality disorder are able to more effectively manage their issues. The therapy for TC is usually located in a residential setting which clients are in for on a regular basis for 1-4 days.

Apart from the group and individual sessions that are part of TC the program also requires patients to take part in other activities to enhance confidence and social skills. The activities are things like performing household chores, preparing dinners and meals playing games, and take part in leisure activities. Therapeutic communities also bring everyone who attends regular community meetings , where people who have different mental health issues meet to discuss their issues and concerns in the community.

One of the most distinctive aspects in the therapy community approach for treatment is the fact that it's operated democratically. Staff, as well as all members can voice their opinion regarding how TC's ought to be managed. In fact, they may even vote on whether that a person should or shouldn't be accepted into the community. That means, even if a therapist believes that a therapeutic group is the best treatment for someone suffering from the disorder known as borderline personality, it does not mean that they'll be allowed entry. A set of guidelines on acceptable conduct is outlined in every TC since they establish restrictions, such as the restriction on alcohol consumption and violence against oneself and others in the community. Anyone who violates the rules are likely to be removed from the TC.

While a therapeutic community is among the most well-known methods of treatment for those suffering from BPD There isn't enough evidence to determine if a TC can be effective for everyone. This is especially true for those with BPD who struggle to adhere to the rules of a TC since they can be very strict in their guidelines.

Self-Care

In during the process of treatment patients usually receive an address that they can dial in case they believe they are experiencing a serious crisis. This can happen when patients suffering from BPD have severe symptoms or episodes and are more susceptible to suicide or self-harm. The number could be referred to community mental health professionals or social workers or other medical experts. Depending on the region there is a crisis resolution is also a possibility as they specialize in providing care for those suffering from serious mental health problems. They often assist patients who require hospitalization for suicide attempts.

People suffering with borderline personality disorder typically discover that speaking to someone about the issues they're experiencing will help them to get out of their misery. Certain instances, though uncommon, might require medications like tranquilizers that can help calm your mood. Such medications are typically prescribed for seven days to help stabilize the moods.

Borderline personality disorder sufferers are advised to join support groups in order to receive social support from others who are experiencing similar experiences like they do. Support groups can help for moral support by sharing thoughts and emotions. Patients can also practice strategies for coping and learn to manage their emotions with people they meet in those support meetings. They've been shown to be a vital component in helping those with BPD improve their skills as they build healthy relationships with others and ultimately reducing the symptoms they experience in the long run.

If you're who suffers from BPD and you are also suffering from BPD, you might be struggling to take better treatment of yourself. But, people diagnosed with BPD must take the initiative to be more attentive to their own health as symptoms can be made worse if they neglect self-care.

Self-care is about taking part in activities that encourage wellbeing and relaxation. This includes exercising regularly and sleep, taking your prescribed medications from your physician, eating healthy food, and managing stress in a healthy way. The people who take good health care of themselves are less likely to suffer from psychiatric issues.

diseases, and that makes self-care essential for all. This is particularly important for those affected by BPD as it could not just aggravate the symptoms, it could also cause more difficult recovery.

Many people are prone to underestimating the importance of sleep when it comes to self-care.

Medication

Some doctors are of the opinion that medication can be beneficial for the treatment of patients with BPD, however other doctors do not agree. There is currently no licensed medication for treating BPD. However, certain types of treatment have proved effective in relieving symptoms for certain individuals.

Typically, selective serotonin receptor inhibitors (SSRI) are usually the first type of medication given to patients. They are intended to decrease anxiety, depression, impulsivity suicidal behaviors, suicidal thoughts as well as anxiety among those suffering from mental health issues.

Anti-depressants as well as anxiety pills can be beneficial to ease symptoms, particularly in the event of a crisis or an emergency. The most commonly used types of antidepressants that are prescribed to those suffering from borderline personality disorder are Prozac, Zoloft, Nardil, Wellbutrin, and Effexor. However, this type of medication is not recommended to use for a long time, mainly because anxiety and depression are usually temporary symptoms that can appear and go in the course of the various stresses within a person's daily life.

Antipsychotics can also have a positive impact on patients, even if they do not suffer from BPD. They can reduce hostility, paranoia and anger and impulsivity among patients with BPD. The most commonly used antipsychotic drugs are Haldol, Clozaril, Risperdal, Seroquel, and Zyprexa.

Mood stabilizers are a different kind of medication that is utilized to treat the symptoms of BPD. They are very effective in dealing with mood swings, impulsivity as well as the extreme emotional changes that are caused by BPD. The most commonly used mood stabilizers are Lithobid, Depakote, Tegretol and Lamictal. A medication that is specifically designed to decrease anxiety is known as anxiolytics and are also prescribed to treat BPD. Anxiolytics are often prescribed to people suffering from BPD however, there is not enough evidence to support the effectiveness of these medications for treating BPD in general. In actual fact there have been instances when certain anxiolytics, also known as benzodiazepines, have been shown to increase manifestations of BPD in people who are not BPD sufferers. The most common types of anxiolytics prescribed to treat BPD sufferers comprise Valium, Xanax, Ativan, Klonopin, and Buspar.

Before deciding to take medication from a doctor it is important to discuss any adverse effects in detail. If the effects appear unnatural, other types of treatment may be considered, particularly in the event that the adverse effects exceed the benefits. The medications used

to treat borderline personality disorder could differ in the form of medication. The most frequent side effects are as follows:
Antidepressants:
Headache
Insomnia
A decreased appetite
Sedation
Sexual dysfunction
Gain in weight
Mood stabilizers:
Acne
Tremors
Weight loss
Gastrointestinal distress
Antipsychotics:
Akathisia
Dry mouth
Gain in weight
Sexual dysfunction
Sedation
Anti-anxiety:
Fatigue
Sleepiness
Mental slowness
Memory issues

Lack of coordination

How Do You Know What Medication is Working

If you begin taking medications to treat borderline personality disorder, it will cause physical and emotional changes. If the medication is working as it should first thing you will be able to notice is a significant change in how you handle situations. While this change can be subtle and gradual, some people benefit from medications at a different pace in comparison to others. Actually, the positive effects are rarely noticeable unless they've been occurring for a long time. It is also typical for others to

Notice the changes in your emotional reaction before you notice observe the changes in your emotional response, and you might want to ask those you typically hang out with about any changes.

Chapter 11: Practice Mindfulness

There's no way you can master something new without any kind of instruction or guidance. Imagine being handed the keys to the keys to a Ferrari and are required to drive it through very heavy traffic, and you've never been on a road in your entire life. This wouldn't go in a good way. The same is true with mindfulness. If it were an issue of saying to you, "Go forth and be aware," then I had better end this book since there's no other thing to do. Don't worry. I'm not going leave you in the dark.

The fundamental principle to Dialectical Behavioral Therapy's philosophy is the practice of mindfulness. What we'll do is look at all the actions you have to take to be mindful. It's not enough to be aware that it's beneficial. I'd like to equip you with the information that you require to help you save yourself.

You might be somewhat skeptical of this. Maybe more than a couple of times, you've thought about putting this book away as you consider it hard to imagine that just developing a mindfulness-based skill could be the only thing you require to transform your life. It's not uncommon to see BPD sufferers to be skeptical about the whole concept. In a situation as complicated as BPD is it possible that someone could ever suggest something so straightforward and simple as mindfulness? What is "mindfulness" actually mean? Mindful? It's tempting to think that it's a religious hoax that is being promoted by Buddhists as a result, and you should not pay any attention. There's no way that to solve all your issues solved with just breathing, and you think. All of these are logical ideas.

It's normal to raise a eyebrow in disbelief about the whole idea even when you don't know what it means to be mindful or even how to begin with it all in the first place.

Once you have a clear idea of what you should do, it is easier for you to take on the idea. However, it isn't enough. It's not enough to be a powerhouse. It's the application of knowledge that gives you everything you need. Even if you are familiar with the mechanics does not mean that you know how to use it. The only way you can truly be able to know is to put into practice the things you know. When I say practice, I don't suggest that you try it just once or twice. You should be consistently consistent with your mindfulness practices. That's how to get the most benefit and improve your performance. It's similar to exercising. You can't hope that every day to reverse years of bad eating habits and a lazy lifestyle. You must continue to work consistently. You must keep working the same muscles repeatedly to make them stronger and stronger. To maintain these muscles in good shape, keep working out as a part of your daily routine. Similar to mindfulness.

The majority of people with BPD are prone to short-term measures such as cutting or reckless behaviour and many other similar things. But the problem is that these measures do not work over the long term. The satisfaction you feel for a moment will only last a few minutes and, in the future, you'll cause yourself or another individual irreparable injury. What's the solution? Mindfulness. When you practice mindfulness, you can experience lasting peace and tranquility. There is a more efficient solution that will benefit you in all situations. It'll take some time and effort and you'll have to be patient but, at the end of the day it will be worth it.

Laying the groundwork

You're likely trying to figure out what frequency and how often you should be mindful. Because you're only getting started it's recommended to begin by practicing for 15 to 20 minutes per day. It's easy to split it into two times one at the beginning of the day and the other at the conclusion.

As you become more comfortable with the routine, you may start adding the time you spend in your practice sessions every day. We'll cover methods to be conscious throughout your daily routine, however we're going to discuss the basics of deciding on a time every day for more concentrated, formal session. This is crucial since being intentional about it can be the sole way to improve your mindfulness. Another thing to note is that regardless of how proficient you get in your mindfulness it is essential that you continue to practice every day.

It is not a requirement. Choose a time comfortable for you and stick to it. If you feel exhausted after a long day, then it's likely that you should be doing your practice in the afternoon, or early in the morning. If you need to begin your day early and have lots to accomplish in order to get your kids ready for school, you may want to think about practicing at night or in the morning. It's your choice. It's up to you to create a habit of it and keep in mind that the only way that habits can be created is through repetition. Make the effort do to make it happen. Make yourself a note in a place you'll keep track of to help you keep track of it, or set an alarm on your phone.

For many people it is beneficial to meditate at a particular spot each time. As I mentioned earlier it isn't necessary to do it, but it can make sense to create a sacred space to practice the practice. In the end, however you'll be able to meditate wherever you happen to be.

Another issue that afflicts people who are brand new to mindfulness is the best posture or position they should take. Should they sit , stand or do something else? There are many various mindfulness techniques. Some of them, you'll have to sit down in some cases, while for others you'll have to move around. It is not necessary to do the lotus pose when you feel it is may be difficult for your knees.

If you're doing a seated meditation, it is recommended to sit in a position where your chest is wide and your arms off of your chest. It is also important to ensure that your lower part is securely and evenly placed upon the floor. Select a chai that lets you sit comfortably. If you require a few pillows to help support your back, you can utilize them. Be sure that your feet are on the ground, but firmly and equally. Don't cross your ankles, or cross your legs. Your shoulders should be straight and straight. Don't slump over. Your arms can be resting on the lap. If you'd like turning your palms up. The most important aspect of this practice is to be mindful of your posture when you sit. Once you've learned how to sit, you'll be able to work on it while keeping the eyes wide.

Controlling Your Mind

The more you work on mindfulness more, you'll realize that your mind is yours. You're in more control of it. At this moment I can understand why you'd believe this is a difficult task. However, it's true! If you are able to practice it, you'll discover that you're not your emotions and thoughts but something else.

The DBT space there is a phenomenon called"the emotional mind. This means that your emotions control the thoughts you make. If you suffer from BPD it's like you're always being tossed around by intense emotions which seem out of control. You are able to accept these feelings, but with devastating effects. Every time you reflect at your actions, it is difficult to be sure why you came to the point at which you behaved the way you did. The inability to focus can cause you to change your mind due to the influence of your emotions, this is why you fail to adhere to the promises you've made to your self and others. You end up destroying relationships that you cherish and making statements that you are not really saying.

In the majority of cases most people don't realize how prevalent thoughts are. We rarely think about our thoughts because we were not taught to think like that. That's where mindfulness is able to help to help us again. If your mind isn't well-trained, it could cause you to suffer a lot of pain and heartache, without realizing it. As a pendulum swings it swings between one extreme and the other. It's possible to get so immersed within your head that you pay too focus on specific thoughts, or you worry until you become obsessed and cannot think beyond the horizon. Whatever the case, you do not focus on your thinking habits. It's almost like you believe that things happen by themselves and you have no control over how you react. It's not necessary to tell you that the extremes of one or the other could create problems, and even pain. Mindfulness can increase your the areas of awareness, curiosity and focus. This is the way to be in control of your mind and get rid of the habits of thinking you've developed.

The Need for Curiosity as well as Awareness

If you're not able to develop your focus, and you're not interested in life then you'll find yourself stuck in your routines. Routines might help you to avoid the pain that you experience but, ultimately they can hold you in a rut and can lead to the discomfort in the future. It is never a good idea to avoid your feelings and thoughts.

You must focus on your thoughts. This means that you should take a moment every now and again and take a glance at your thoughts. What speed or how slow are your thoughts? Is your mind a chaotic mess or well-organized? Are they loving and caring or angry and bitter? What is it exactly that you're contemplating?

The goal of mindfulness is taking control of your thoughts as well as your thinking processes, and, by extension your feelings. When you're attentive to what you are thinking about, the peace and calm that you experience will be a hundred times greater. It can be hard for you to accept that awareness could assist you in achieving all this, especially if you've never tried previously, however I can assure that it will work.

The Practice

While you are practicing be aware of the way your body and mind feel. This will allow you to learn what that you could do in order to reduce your pain and suffering caused by your thoughts and emotions. In the DBT space, these activities are known as "what" as well as "how" abilities"what" and "how" skills "what" is the action you do to stay in the present and "how" being the way you do it "how" is how you approach it.

You should try the exercises you'll learn by this text at least once. You'll require a notebook to write notes about your experience following each practice. It is likely that certain of the exercises are more beneficial to you than other. However do not commit to the ones you're currently using without trying all of them, to see which ones work for you and what does not. The objective isn't getting you to enjoy the method, but rather to inspire you to be more curiousand offer your brain a challenge.

I'd like to mention that there are days when you'll feel like your training was a bit better than the other days. This doesn't mean you're not doing well. It's just how it is. You're having a blast with your routine; the next day, you're finding the same routine to be challenging. The benefit of mindfulness is that the experience of it is ever changing, never static.

Another thing I want to be aware of is that your mind is likely to wander. You should be comfortable with this fact. If you find that your mind is in a different direction Do not get angry on yourself. It's actually a sign of an improvement! Just bring your attention back to your goal regardless of what it is. Every moment your mind wanders and you return it you'll become more proficient at maintaining your focus. Keep in mind that your brain is just like muscles. This is the way it becomes stronger.

The Intentional Power of Intention

It is impossible to practice mindfulness without the intention. Intention is a wonderful thing because when you are able to do things without thinking about it, then when you are focused, then you could effectively do it in a mindful manner. Intention is when you decide to be attentive to something with a particular objective in your mind. This means that you can brush your teeth as usual and your mind is on autopilot, thinking about mortgages and bills and mortgages, or you could spend your time paying attention to the ways you brush, how your mouth feels and the list goes on. You are aware of the need to consider ways to pay the bills, but you return your focus to the simple task of cleaning your teeth. As you brushyour teeth, your mind may wander away. If this happens it, you can come back to your brushing. This can be done in any task you perform on a regular basis such as walking, driving, doing dishes or washing cleaning your clothes. This is how you can infuse mindfulness into your everyday activities.

There's a myth that the entire purpose of mindfulness is having a an unchanging mind. That's impossible. There will always be thoughts in your mind. That's the purpose that your brain performs. What is mindfulness? It's deliberate decision to bring your focus back to the task at hand every moment the mind drifts. The goal isn't to keep your thoughts secluded and empty.

Choose, Commit, and Succeed

If you choose to become more aware, you need to constantly remind yourself of what you've chosen to accomplish and the reason behind it. It is important that at the beginning, you're confident about the fact that you'll need to pay attention to you've picked to accomplish be it making dishes or cleaning your car. Make yourself promise yourself that you'll complete this in a mindful manner, and your brain gets a signal that it must focus on the task at hand. When you make this commitment you're more likely to be successful.

A Different Method for Each Day

All you have to do is to make a change to at minimum one thing you routinely do every day, and only for one week. If you're habitual of getting up on the left Try getting up onto the right side. Do you typically unlock doors using the dominant hand? Make a commitment to use the opposite hand. It's about trying something new for a specified amount of time and giving all attention to the procedure.

Watching

Another skill that practicing mindfulness can provide is observation. It will be easier to be aware of the thoughts you think about and how you feel. In DBT it is referred to by the "observe" capability.

When you practice mindful observation, there's no need to be looking in the hope of judging or defining things. It's simply about taking note of your experience and not trying to put it to a specific category. The moment you are in is experienced completely, using the fullest of your awareness. The difficulty here isn't the issue of labelling anything.

In the majority of cases we go about everything we do, without paying any at it, and this is the reason we often miss important bits of information that can improve our lives. When you begin to be aware to what that you've gotten used to will be apparent to you. This is particularly beneficial for people suffering from BPD because a significant portion of the issue that is associated with BPD is the unthinking automatic responses that can cause inhuman suffering. If you discover that you have some person or something who you respond with anger, once you become more conscious and aware, you'll realize that it's a natural reaction that you've become accustomed to due to repeated exposure, making it a routine. You'll soon realize that you have the option of choosing. You may choose to react differently, in the same manner you would have started laces on your left shoe prior to your left during your mindfulness exercises.

Another superpower mindfulness gives one is being able to observe your emotions during the initial stages prior to them blossoming into full-blown. When you can tell you're experiencing anger or sadness before you completely surrender to your emotions and you no longer think that your emotions "just occur" in your life. You'll realize that you're in charge. You'll be aware that at any moment in time, you are able to change your feelings. Don't get overwhelmed by emotions that are intense.

Just watching is a great method of calming your mind. This can be quite challenging particularly since you do not require words. We are prone to assigning terms to everything we see. To test this, go outside with yourself, taking in the sights and sounds without assigning any terms to these. Beginning it will not be simple. Imagine seeing a red rose without needing to call the flower "a Red Rose" in your head? It's not an easy task at first however, as time passes, you will get better at it. When you observe your surroundings without judgment or labeling the part of your brain that is responsible for thinking will slow down and go to sleep. This is the part of your brain that is hyperactive when you're stressed or anxious. out. Simply watching at, observing, and paying attention can calm your mind and body tremendously. It is about moving from a state that is characterized by action performing, thinking, and doing into a state of beingunaffected by external or internal factors.

Chapter 12: Learning To Cope Skills Toolkit.

Everyone has good days as well as we all experience bad days. The experience of either is more intense if you suffer from BPD. A set of coping strategies should be developed to enable you to quickly discover ways to handle bad (or multiple) occasions. Think of it as the Coping Skills Toolkit. This doesn't need to be a tangible toolkit. Most of the information are conceptual However, you can make your own list of "items" that you can put into this kit and take it around on your person. If you're overwhelmed by emotions, it is difficult to recall the skills you use to cope or think clearly about any topic. If you keep your list in your pocket you can easily find ways to manage your emotions. Here's an outline of the kinds of things you could add.

Grounding skills. Similar to the ones mentioned above, they can help you focus on the immediate mental and physical stimuli. Utilize auditory or visual stimuli to help you forget the immediate negative emotions. Take note of the sounds that surround you, not only the obvious ones, but any sound you hear. Be aware of the ways that they fluctuate - for instance, on a busy street, you'll hear the rumble of traffic, the snippets of conversations and the sound of birdsong (perhaps) as well as the sound of construction activities. So long as you're safe, take a moment to lose yourself in the sounds of the world around you for a while.

Journal-keeping. This is a technique that many who suffer from BPD are able to use for creating triggers, evaluating feelings and making lists of both pros and cons. Make your writing expressive and express whatever you wish to and say everything you feel. Sometimes, simply writing this way can rid you of negative thoughts without being a danger to others! Do not worry about the small things such as spelling, grammar, or even understanding. Write as long as you'd like!

Positive actions. Find activities that will alleviate your negative feelings. Doing the dishes, cleaning the oven or just sitting down and knitting! In reality any activity that is repetitive and requires focus is an great for managing your emotions and reduce the intense feelings you experience from these.

These are just the fundamental ideas to add to your Coping Skills Toolkit. They could be helpful for anyone, however you could also need to come up with your own strategies to manage the fluctuations and peaks of BPD. The most important thing to make is to list them out take them with you and make as comprehensive an inventory as you can. Find things you can perform at home within the comfort in your home (knitting for instance) as well as ones are suitable for when you're on the move or working (simple mindfulness, for instance). Make sure you have a mix of both so that no matter the circumstance, you will be able to find an easy coping strategy which is suitable for the circumstance.

After you've compiled your list of skills, work on them; Not all the abilities are going to come naturally to you and you might have to keep working on certain skills until they are. When you practice, you're strengthening the skills you already have within your brain and they'll be readily available when you need they. In time, you'll realize that your default response to stressful situations is to utilize one of your new abilities instead of taking self-destructive actions as you did previously. This, as we mentioned at the beginning in the text, will be the moment when your BPD will start to become less of a concern on a regular basis and you'll be on your way towards recovery.

BPD and Self-Esteem

In the majority of instances of BPD you'll notice that self-esteem problems are an aspect of life! Many times BPD develops in the adolescent years and is due to the abuse or neglect. This is often a result of emotional neglect , and is an outcome of being told that one's opinions or feelings aren't valid. The people who have low self-esteem usually believe that they have nothing to offer other people or to the world at large. There are many methods that can help you build or restore self-esteem, and in this article, we'll explore some of the basic strategies. Although these are the most basic, it is important to use each of them on a regular basis. Building a sense of self-worth isn't easy and may take a considerable amount of time. These tasks and exercises are not too difficult to be completed quickly, frequently and aren't too difficult or burdensome. When you are successful in every one (frequently and frequently) you'll be able to build an enduring foundation to feel confident of self-worth. Also, you're able to tackle larger tasks or projects that expand on this.

Positive Self-Talk. How would you describe yourself to yourself? "I'm as a fool"? "I'm an utter waste of space"? "I'm not worthy of knowing"? It's not uncommon to feel this way at times, but these thoughts don't increase your self-esteem. It's normal when things happen to you to make use of this type of "self-talk" especially for those suffering from BPD. Positive self-talk involves repositioning these thoughts. Did you miss an important appointment? "I've got it wrong it happens!" might be a better way to express yourself. "Oh that's fine, this isn't the final word" is another great one , and it's also real. To date, no one alive (or deceased) has committed an error that led to that result, and likelihood is that if it occurs, it won't your fault. Do your best to be kind to yourself.

Take Charge. You don't need to be in charge of huge things to have a positive impact on the way you live. Clean up a drawer, arrange an office filing system, and redesign a space. Make a decision that allows you to plan and then complete the task in a straightforward manner. Take it step-by-step and you will see your achievements appear each step. It is possible to consider bigger initiatives (like jumping bungees or other challenges that you face personally) when you're confident however, small steps are the best place to begin.

Participate in a charity or volunteer work. It's extremely beneficial, since it's about helping others and feeling fulfilled. It can help you build a sense of self-worth and have value to the world, and it will also allow you to be out and about with others. This is not easy but making new acquaintances and broadening your horizons could give a huge increase in self-esteem.

Then, you should attend your sessions with a therapist. The entire book is intended to provide the reader simple, fundamental ideas to help you manage each day that you are suffering from BPD. But, therapy sessions with a professional will be the place where you can get the most benefit and they'll be able to will not only assist you build confidence and demonstrate that you can overcome the disease as well as aid your ultimate recovery.

Last Words

BPD is a common affliction however, among all the mental or emotional problems it's one with the highest chance of long-term and durable recovery. It could take years for a complete recovery however it is crucial to establish this goal right from the beginning. If you have BDP or were recently diagnosed It's crucial to keep in mind that emotions aren't, in and of themselves, harmful. They are an integral part of our psychological makeup, and vital in our everyday lives. Understanding how to manage these emotions, manage their intensity and deal with intense emotions can be difficult, but it's not a difficult task!

Chapter 13: What Can You Do To Improve Social Relations

There aren't many guidelines that can aid you in making an impression. Take a look at the five points laid below and you'll have an possibility of connecting with many people in a social group.

Lights for the start

When they first meet or getting more acquainted with someone there are many people who will bombard the other person with a series of "talk with fashion" questions. (Where are you from? What are you doing? What do you think you would like to see from to do it? And and so further.). This kind of discussion isn't just exhausting; it's extremely awkward to respond to a flood of inquiries from someone who doesn't even have the slightest clue about.

Instead of kicking out the door open with these types of questions If you're in the ideal position to get this show off the road with a conversation that is light and without content. For instance, you could comment on something that's happening in your life. On the other hand, you could you can open up by a bit of playful pushing (simply be sure to keep smiling when you're trying to get her attention to let her know you're not joking). If you're not sure if you're feeling the conversation, you could usually begin by giving an acknowledgement - perhaps on something they're wearing that you think is interesting.

Assemble affinity

In every social gathering, no matter whether it's business or personal, or a casual meeting with a girl in an establishment, it's essential to build a bond. What are the best ways to do this? Start by using the "I" view in your discussions about your thoughts, feelings and conclusion. As an example instead of declaring "b-ball is the most enjoyable game ever" like it's some kind of goal certainty, you could say "I am a huge fan of the game of b-ball" and then perhaps talk about the benefits you gain from it, and what makes you enjoy it.

It may seem like an unnoticeable contrast, but using this "I" perspective lets people see the inner world of your mind - your thoughts, emotions and more. Furthermore by giving people this more enlightened look, it allows them to see that you are someone that has similar feelings to them. This creates a strong bond and makes them feel more connected with you.

Provide services

A certain attitude can aid you greatly in social interactions. It can be difficult to acquire every now and again However, in the event that people would want to be a part of your group regardless of what is anticipated. That is the view of a company. When you make connections, don't expect to "get" something. Do not meet a girl just trying to get a contact number, or meet with a VIP business person to ensure he'll show improvements. If you're looking to establish an established relationship with this young lady in order for her to be able to date you, or the VIP wants to make an effort to get you an occupation, begin with a positive attitude. Try to make the girl a memorable meeting and brighten her day. Help the VIP to overcome whatever problem they may face. If you keep your focus on constantly giving, without a desire to receive anything as a result many people will feel pressured to contribute. The young lady you are looking for will have to give you her phone number and that VIP is expected to assist you in getting an amazing job. It's not going to happen all the all the time, however in the long run, focusing on what you can provide instead of the amount you can earn will yield huge earnings.

You are ineffective

In almost every type of social connection, people are worried about what they are trampled upon. It's amazing when someone lets them know that it's okay to take off the "social curtain". It means they no longer have to stress about trying in vain to "look nice" and be a part of it with their appearance, and be who they are and still be recognized.

A great way to make this entrance open and let people know it's okay to relax, unwind and be yourself is to take the lead and let yourself be in charge. For instance, if you're unsure regarding some aspect (your weight, the way you're dressed, how nervous you are...) Don't try to cover it up and hope that nobody takes note. Instead, shine a bright shine on the issue. Make it a point to highlight it and belittle you for doing it (simply do not be a natural snarky troll). Making a point of highlighting your flaws and laughing at them will assist others to relax contemplating their flaws. To add a little additional, it is an excellent method to create an incredibly deep connection.

Be positive and keep it that way

There isn't a type of social cooperation that is modified by a negative state of mind. The more positive and constructive you are when working with others as well as your interactions with others, the more people will be happy to work with you. All things considered, the way you behave can be infective. In addition in the event you need to remain pleasant and constructive in a group you will rub off your friends. Additionally, they'll appreciate being around you.

Effective Communication - Enhancing your Social Skills

Being able to build strong relationships with others can greatly reduce pressure and stress in your life. Actually, improving your social interaction is related to better mental health overall, as having great friends can serve as "support" for feelings of sadness and depression. However the case for certain people, their stress can lead to their inability to deal with social interactions, and hinder their connections from developing. This is especially true when you're feeling anxious and desperately need to meet friends, but feel in too much pain to think about it or aren't sure how to make connections with other people.

Unfortunately, one result of keeping the distance of a separation from social situations is that you don't have the opportunity to:

Build your confidence in interacting with other people.

Build strong interpersonal skills that will allow to make connections that are effective

For instance, in the possibility that you are hesitant to go to gatherings or taking someone to go out Your lack of experience and also a lack of confidence can make it much more difficult to determine how you will handle these scenarios (like how to dress, what to say and so on.). Most of the time, people have the necessary skills, but aren't able to demonstrate the confidence to use these skills. Practice can build confidence and increase your ability to communicate.

Why are Communication Skills Essential?

These skills are essential to establish (and maintaining) connections and to build an effective social group of people. They also assist you in managing your personal needswhile being mindful of the needs of other people. People aren't born to the world with exceptional interpersonal skills; as with other talents, they're learned through trial and error and repeated exercises.

Three areas of correspondence you may need to practice are:

Non-VERBAL CORRESPONDENCE

Discuss APTITUDE DISCUSSION

The emphasis

Note: Naturally there are many ways to write compelling letters and you might require more explicit help in particular areas (for instance, figuring out how to manage conflict intro skills, how to give critique, etc.). For more explicit help in cases where it's not too difficult, look up this "Prescribed readings" list at the end of this course.

Non-Verbal Communication

The majority of the information we share with each other is non-verbal. What you say to people through your eyes or non-verbal communications are just remarkable as the words you say using words. When you feel anxious you could behave in ways that are designed to avoid speaking to other people. For instance, you could avoid eye-to-eye communication or converse in a calm manner. The point is that you're doing everything you can to avoid having to transmit, but to avoid being considered unpopular by other people. In any event your non-verbal communication and style of speech sends powerful messages to others about you:

State of passion (for instance, eagerness or anxiety,)

The way you think about the target audience (for instance, apathy, anger)

Information about the topic

Sincerity (do do you possess a mysterious plan?)

In the event that you're keeping a distance of eye to eye contact and avoiding other people and speaking in a discreet manner in a quiet manner, you're likely to be delivering, "Avoid me!" or "Don't engage me!" or "Don't talk to me!" the message you want to convey.

Discussion Skills

The most likely test for someone who is prone to social tension is starting conversations and sustaining them. It's not unusual to be at war with one another when trying to engage in casual conversation as it's not in all cases easy to think about remarks. This is especially evident when you're feeling discontent. However, some edge people continue to be agitated for hours, which could have an impact on other people.

Self-assuredness

Self-assured correspondence is a genuine communication of one's desires, feelings and needs in relation to the needs and feelings of another. When you speak clearly your message, you are non-compromising and uncritical and you are accountable for your actions.

If you're in a social situation that's tense it is possible that you will have difficulty communicating your thoughts and thoughts in a way that is clear. Self-assurance skills can be challenging to master, especially since being self-assured could result in a reluctance to follow the way you normally accomplish things. In other words, you may be apprehensive about conflict, always be a good sport to the group and refrain from making assertions. In this way, you might have developed an unrestrained manner of correspondence. However you could be aiming to rule over other people and have built an effective correspondence style.

As it happens using a clear and concise manner of correspondence has numerous benefits. For instance, it could aid you in relating with people more effectively without a lot of anxiety and anger. Additionally, it provides you with more control over your own life, and reduces feelings of being in powerlessness. In addition, it gives other people to lead their lives.

Chapter 14: What To Eliminate

Anxiety

Whatever function you are playing in your life being able to manage and express your emotions is certain to play a significant part. Also, you must be able to comprehend how to interpret, respond, and react with the appropriate emotions that people around you also feel. Imagine how difficult it would feel if you could not tell the time when one of your closest acquaintances was sad or when one of your colleagues was angry at you. If you're not just capable of controlling and expressing your own emotions, but also understand and interpret the emotions of others you're considered to have emotional intelligence.

In a nutshell the term "emotional intelligence" refers to the ability to sense the impact of, manage, and assess emotions, regardless of whether they are your own emotions or ones that another person is experiencing. Some people have higher emotional intelligence and can manage the emotions they feel in a variety of situations, while also reacting to the feelings of others who are around them. However certain people are lacking emotional intelligence. They are people who be ablaze at anything and are unable to take the emotions of others into account.

Let's examine the differences between an individual with emotional intelligence and another who does not. The first one is one who accepts life as it is. They know that the majority of the times whenever things do go wrong it's out of their control, rather than viewing it as if the world is attacking them directly. They are not often upset particularly over small issues and are aware of the appropriate moments to express their feelings.

Furthermore that, this person reacts well to what others feel. When a coworker walks in and starts shouting on them, they do not immediately respond. It is clear that some thing might be bothering the person and step in to assist or fix the issue that is the root of the issue. If one of their friends has a bad day They talk about the issues and help them get better.

Let's now take a look at the second person. This person has a tough managing their emotions. If they're upset over something, they can be angry with others (whether it's the someone else's fault or not) and they can cry easily and may experience anxiety. People who are upset often have an idea that the whole universe is against them. tiny things, the ones which don't really matter are enough to trigger their anger.

When it comes down to how they respond to others, it's only an idea. They do not pay attention to the opinions of their acquaintances and consider how they personally affected by the events. If someone else is angry at them, they believe they're being treated unfairly. The entire world is against them and people don't get it.

The first person we have met is one who is a person with a high degree in emotional intelligence. The person is able to identify and manage their emotions. They are able to discern the other people's emotions who are around them. The other person has a lower level of emotional intelligence. They're constantly angry about every single thing, and may do not know why they have the emotions that they are, but aren't paying at the emotions of other people. Of obviously, there are variations in between the two extremes. knowing your degree of intelligence could be crucial in helping to grow.

Many believe that it is possible to increase your emotional intelligence through laborious work. However, there are those who believe this is an inherent characteristic that you're born with, which makes it difficult and even impossible to alter. There's likely to be some truth in both schools of thinking. We all have an inherent level of emotional intelligence that we can enhance and nurture or let to a point of no return through a lack of use.

The four components of emotional intelligence

There are four primary elements that will define your emotional intelligence. They include:

Perceiving emotions: the first thing you have to do to comprehend emotions is to understand how to detect them accurately. This could include learning to discern nonverbal signals, such as body language and facial expressions.

* Thinking with emotions: The next thing to do is to use your emotions to increase cognitive stimulation. It can be difficult initially however, emotions can help identify what we're watching and responding too, and we should be aware of this in order to discover more about ourselves.

Understanding emotions: There are a variety of meanings that be associated with the emotions we feel. For instance, if you notice that someone is unhappy, it is possible to look behind and consider what is causing them to feel how they feel. The boss might be angry at you over your work due to a dispute in front of their supervisor, had a fight with their wife, received a speeding ticket or for any number of other motives. A person with an elevated level of emotional intelligence is capable of recognizing this.

* Managing your emotions: Next is the ability to successfully handle your feelings. You should be able to control your emotions, determine the appropriate response, and then act in a way that is an integral element of your emotional management.

There are many ways you can gauge the level of your psychological intelligence. There are a variety of tests that you can do to determine this, however, it's possible to identify your own emotional intelligence , and improve it with hard work and determination. When you learn to recognize your emotions, the reasons leading them, and then the right response to the current situation You can enhance your emotional intelligence in a shorter period of time than you think.

Then why do you need to focus your efforts on your emotional intelligence? There are many scenarios in your daily life where an increased degree of emotional intelligence could have a significant impact. For instance at work. People with more emotional intelligence are those who are more productive because they choose jobs they love as well as work better in interacting with colleagues, convince others to agree with their views and avoid conflict. Think about how these abilities could be helpful at work regardless of whether you're trying to get ahead or keep up-to-date. Everyone can benefit from brushing up on these abilities to be more effective at work.

Another important area where you can realize the benefits from working with emotional intelligence is when it comes to relationships, whether they are in your relationship with a spouse, your family members, or your colleagues. Everyone you interact with is likely to feel their own emotions and being able to identify them and react in the appropriate manner can make it much easier to come to be a good friend. When conflicts do arise you'll be able to manage your emotions to avoid a larger fracas that isn't necessary, no matter the type of relationship you're trying to build.

Conclusion

The process of separating from a partner that is this kind of thing isn't straightforward and I'd like to thank you for choosing to act in response to the situation. This program isn't by any way going to transform your life in a single day - it isn't an instant fix. But if you regularly utilize the tools I have gave you, certain you will witness dramatic positive changes in all areas that you live. I'd like to leave you with this famous quote by Ghandi:

"Your beliefs are your thoughts."

Your thoughts turn into words,

Your words are what you do,

Your actions are your habits

Your actions transform into your values

Your values become your destiny."